As THEY SEE IT

THE DEVELOPMENT OF THE
AFRICAN AIDS DISCOURSE

Published by
Adonis & Abbey Publishers Ltd
P.O. Box 43418
London
SE11 4XZ
http://www.adonis-abbey.com

First Edition, April 2005

British Library Cataloguing-in-Publication Data
A catalogue record for this book is available from the British Library

ISBN 0-905068-07-7

Cover Design: Heather Churchill

Printed and bound in Great Britain by Lightning Source UK Ltd.

As They See It

The Development of the African AIDS Discourse

By

Raymond Downing, MD

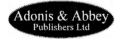

To J.N.K. Mugambi

As They See It
The Development of the African AIDS Discourse

Table of Contents

Preface and Acknowledgements

News items about AIDS in Africa repeatedly find their way to the front pages of newspapers in Europe and North America. In most of them, the same players and themes recur: the UN and its statistics of doom, the pharmaceutical companies and their profits, the activists and their passion, and the hapless African governments lost in poverty and corruption. Little is reported about what African leaders and scholars think about their own epidemic—except, of course, South African President Thabo Mbeki, and most reports have vilified him.

Another story emerges, however, when we look more closely at what Mbeki has actually said about AIDS (rather than how he has been interpreted), and when we consider what other Africans have said about him. His approach to AIDS is far more helpful than the media have led us to believe. However, the standard by which we judge AIDS programs is the biomedical standard—as it is practiced in the West—rooted in Western ethical assumptions. It is according to this standard and these assumptions that we in the West have written off Mbeki's view of AIDS. More seriously, how the rest of Africa views this epidemic remains mostly hidden from view.

The story of how Africa views AIDS needs to be told, including a reexamination of the Mbeki controversy. In telling this story, I have begun with some of the questions that are on the minds of many in Africa, followed by a review and an analysis of what African scholars working in Africa have said about AIDS. I have made no attempt to be exhaustive, to cover every African conference and scholar and book on AIDS; I have rather tried to be representative, looking at conferences and books and scholars and trends that point to *distinctively* African approaches to the disease. Consequently, there is little here that draws from biomedical research done by Africans, as that research is, to some extent, "culture-blind". What we do with the results of that research, however, has everything to do with culture.

It has been said that Africa sometimes defines itself in response to events that happen to it and how they are viewed in the rest of the world. Indeed, Laurenti Magesa says of the essays that comprise his *Christian Ethics in Africa*, "They themselves were in the main responses or reactions, even if perhaps unconscious, to challenges I encountered listening to others or reading their opinions and stated positions."[1] AIDS is certainly one of those major events happening in Africa, and the way the rest of the world sees this epidemic provides a challenge for thoughtful African response. Examining these responses can be a window into how Africans view themselves and the rest of the world. Consequently, although the subject matter of this book is AIDS, the African reflections come with an invitation to look beyond the specific disease being examined. AIDS is providing the world with an opportunity to see how Africans view health and disease generally.

Some people have challenged me—and I have asked myself— who am I to write this book? Shouldn't the "African view" be written by Africans? Of course—and Africans have written. The problem is that these African views are for the most part not being read by people in the West. Thus, from our perspective, Africa is "silent" about AIDS. Activist physician Paul Farmer says that the poor suffer in silence, but this silence is "imposed from above... For underneath this silence lies the pent-up anger born of innumerable small indignities, and of great and irremediable ones." The same could be said of African academics, ignored by those with enough money to make policy *for* Africa. Farmer's response is to "bear witness" to the suffering of the poor. "Bearing witness is done on behalf of others, for their sake... It needs to be done, but there is no point exaggerating the importance of the deed."[2] My intent is to bear witness to the existence of a serious, well-developed African discourse on AIDS, and to acknowledge the "structural violence", as Farmer calls it, that keeps this discourse from being heard.

Though I am a physician, this is neither a medical text nor is it bound to any of the other academic disciplines. I am not a social science researcher. I am simply a medical doctor who happens to have spent more of my professional life working in Africa than in the US. The only "expertise" I claim is the set of skills needed to be a physician—which includes the ability to listen to a patient's story of their disease, and then organize and record that story in a logical and chronological fashion. This is called the medical history, and when done well should lead to one or several diagnoses. It is this skill of telling a story of a disease that I am relying on as I try to tell the story of the *development* of the discourse of AIDS in Africa.

There is a corollary to this stance. As a physician, it is my job to determine whether or not a person has, for example, pain, and record where and when they have that pain. The question of whether they *ought* to have pain – whether someone with a similar insult would have comparable pain – is an important but separate question. Likewise in recording the development of the discourse of AIDS in Africa, it is not my task to evaluate whether or not Mbeki or any other African *ought* to feel the way they do, nor whether their position is "right" (according to my standard of rightness). If I can expose, and possibly explain, what some Africans are saying about AIDS, and make that intelligible to Western ears, I will be content.

A few final notes on the text: All of my source materials were in English, clearly a limitation for a continent whose writers are equally likely to publish their reflections in French or Arabic. On the other hand, the countries in Africa that have the highest prevalence of AIDS are in eastern and southern Africa, regions where English is the main second language. Once again, this book is not trying to be the *whole* story, but simply a representative story. Regarding language, I have used "the West" to refer to societies based on European culture, including the United States. Most of these places are also wealthy. Similarly, I use "Africa" to mean sub-Saharan or black Africa. I do not assume that all Africans are alike any more than I assume all Westerners are alike; I use the general terms when I am talking about characteristics that many Westerners do share, or many Africans do share.

Regarding the term "AIDS": AIDS is an acronym for Acquired Immune Deficiency Syndrome, and in several countries it has lost its capitals and is called Aids or even aids. I use capitals unless I am quoting someone who doesn't. Some writers routinely call the condition "HIV/AIDS", partly to make the point that HIV is the cause. Others want to emphasize that whereas AIDS is a disease, asymptomatic HIV status is important but different. I agree with all that. But we don't usually call malaria "P. falciparum/malaria"; we don't usually call typhoid "salmonella/typhoid" — even though in both of these cases a person without symptoms can have the infection and can pass it on to others while being asymptomatic. These distinctions may be important in medical papers and public health programs, but are less so when viewing these diseases in their psycho-social-cultural-spiritual contexts. I use "AIDS" when referring to a person who is ill (whether from AIDS or its related infections), and "HIV positive" or "sero-positive" for someone who has the virus (and can transmit it) but is not yet ill.

Non-fiction authors always have sources, and in this book I have chosen to only quote from sources which are in the public domain – books, journals, newspaper articles, and internet sites. I did not find them all alone. Many acquaintances and friends helped me to find these sources and understand what they meant, both in face to face conversation and by email. Others challenged or confirmed, and clarified or modified my thinking, and all, by their involvement, encouraged me:

In Botswana: Prof. Emevo Biakolo (you generously opened several doors), Prof. Nobantu Rasebotsa, and people at the Mennonite Guest House.

In Kenya: Kariuki Thuku, Mosala Mfungisi, Timothy Gachanga, Dr. Haruun Ruun, Dr. Peter Okaalet, Prof. Jesse Mugambi (I hope your perspective will work on me until I get it right), Kennedy Lubisia, Dr. Lumarai Lugaria, Prof. Ruth Muthei James, Prof. Grace Wamue, Prof. Constance Shisanya, Harold Miller (who started me on this journey) and Annetta Miller (for the proverbs in the Afterword), Erna and Larry Lowen-Rudgers (for hospitality and more).

In South Africa: Dr. Neville Jada, Prof. Sam Mhlongo, Phaswane Mpe (who welcomed us to Hillbrow), Bob Phatho and Opa (for confirming there is more than one South African view about Mbeki and AIDS), Joe Bobo, Chris Ntyobile, Vernon, Tineke, Thobo and Amanda Gibberd (for hospitality and more), people at the B&B in Soweto.

In Tanzania: Mosi Kisare (a wonderful teacher), Fr. Laurenti Magesa (another wonderful teacher), Dr. Mark Jacobson and Mama Peter, Pauline, and Mary (you revived our Swahili).

In Uganda: Alex Bogere, , Leo Mmerewoma, Bishop Ochola, Prof. Peter Kanyandago, Prof. Emanuel Katongole (clear thinking and encouragement come together), Prof. Byaruhanga-Akiki, Dave and MaryLou Klassen (for hospitality and more).

In the United States: Prof. Kathryn Herr (who helped liberate information) and Prof. Gary Anderson, Dr. John Shaw, Tim Lind, Prof. Wende Marshall (you are a rare find in the US), Prof. Nancy Scheper-Hughes, Dr. Elizabeth Onjoro, Dr. Ron Pust (unceasing honest encouragement), Prof. Musa Dube, Olabode Ibironke (thank you for extending my list for the fiction chapter), Cindy Patton, Jim Lance (your belief in this project is unforgettable), Elizabeth Downing (research assistant and editor) and my wife Dr. Jan Armstrong, who lived every page with me.

References

---

[1] **Magesa, Laurenti (2002):** *Christians Ethics in Africa,* (Nairobi, Acton Publishers,) p. 1-2.

[2] **Farmer, Paul (2003):** *Pathologies of Power: Health, Human Rights, and the New War on the Poor* (Berkeley, University of California Press,) p. 25-28.

Prologue

Why Is It So Difficult for the West to Hear African voices?

In the Preface to a recent book on AIDS in Africa and the Caribbean, the editors dealt with their lack of inclusion of African voices this way: "The editors are very aware of a major lack in this volume. We do not intend to marginalize or silence the voices of Africans and persons from the Caribbean, either researchers or AIDS victims. We are very conscious that research in Uganda, for example, could not have been done by the anthropologists and historian whose work you will be reading in this volume, were it not for Ugandans' willingness to share their knowledge and views. The two articles by David Serwadda, the clinician who first diagnosed Slim in 1982, are taken by Bond and Vincent as benchmarks in the history of the AIDS epidemic in Uganda."[1]

At first, this seems to be a simple humble recognition of the value of African voices – except that instead of being an introduction to these voices, it is an excuse for not including them. Bond and Vincent apparently do a good enough job in informing us of Serwadda's contribution. We never see it, or any other African contribution, directly. It would have been better to not mention the "major lack in this volume" at all, rather than to point it out and then do nothing about it – effectively marginalizing and silencing the African voices that are not in fact included.

It's a perennial problem. In 1990 several African scholars published *Beyond Hunger in Africa*[2], the results of a 1987 exercise by those scholars to articulate alternative visions for Africa's future. The conventional wisdom then was that Africa was a continent in crisis because of famine; today the crisis is AIDS. The sentiments of the introductory chapter, written in the context of hunger, could apply equally to AIDS. Consider these excerpts:

Perhaps the most tragic aspect of this situation is that the debate about Africa's future is dominated by the

international community. Those who are farthest removed
from African realities – who do not feel the pinch or who
need not take responsibility – are the pace-setters. In fact,
even more than in the past, the prevailing notion is that
Africa cannot move ahead without the aid of the
international community.... As the 'crippled' region of the
world, Africa is largely treated in a paternalistic fashion....
In brief, Africa today suffers in particular because of the
following three shortcomings:
- The image of Africa is one-sided
- Africa's own voice is ignored
- Africa's domestic capacity is neglected. [3]

Some Western scholars agree. Paula Treichler, in *How to Have
Theory in an Epidemic*[4], says "deeply entrenched institutional
agendas and cultural precedents in the First World prevent us from
hearing the story of AIDS in the Third World as a complex
narrative... In concrete terms, we need to forsake, at least part of
the time, the coherent AIDS narrative of the Western professional
and technological agencies and listen instead to multiple sources
about and within the Third World."

Treichler is not alone. A more recent book, *HIV and AIDS in
Africa: Beyond Epidemiology*,[5] recognizes the same problems. When
"biomedical models remain dominant in generating
understandings of AIDS in Africa," there is a "tendency in these
studies to focus on sexual practices devoid of socioeconomic
contexts," consequently ignoring "the social embeddedness of
vulnerability." The larger question in *Beyond Epidemiology* is "how
Africa as well as AIDS has come to be 'known', what knowledge is
privileged, and how it gets deployed. We are concerned, for
example, that dominant interpretations of AIDS are aiding in the
reproduction of problematic colonial and postcolonial African
representations, practices, and social politics." The African scholars
from *Beyond Hunger in Africa* would likely agree. The authors of
Beyond Epidemiology continue:

Perhaps the most visible example of what is at stake in conflicting interpretations of AIDS is still playing out in South Africa. South African President Thabo Mbeki's controversial stance on AIDS as a disease of poverty rather than an epidemic driven by HIV has caused profound consternation among international researchers as well as frustration among physicians and AIDS activists within South Africa (cf. Treatment Action Campaign at www.tac.za.org). While these concerns are more than understandable given Mbeki's refusal to provide antiretrovirals to affected populations, the incontrovertible dominance of biomedical models placing HIV front and center have silenced Mbeki's more insightful statements on poverty's role in creating AIDS in the South African context.

That is a fair introduction to Mbeki – but in this 398 page book it remains only an introduction. Mbeki is not mentioned again in the entire book. His "more insightful statements" remain "silenced". To be sure, there are other African voices in the book – but "the most visible example" is dropped. Why?

Why is it so difficult for the West to hear Mbeki and other African voices?

On one level, concerning Mbeki at least, the answer seems simple. In 2000, Mbeki engaged in extended conversations with scientific "dissidents" from the West, some of whom deny that the virus HIV causes the disease AIDS. Since the vast majority of those working with AIDS accept the link between HIV and AIDS – and since Mbeki was presumably guilty by association with these dissidents – the easiest approach was to ridicule Mbeki, and then dismiss him. While this was a common response in the media several years ago, the sentiment still exists, as shown by an example from a recent issue of a prominent medical journal.

The July 1, 2004 issue of *The New England Journal of Medicine* contained an article looking at, among other things, AIDS in South Africa.[6] The author, Solomon Benatar from the University of Cape Town, said:

The approach of the South African government to HIV and AIDS has been resoundingly criticized within the country and internationally. It has been a disappointment that a new, enlightened democratic government could so arrogantly deny the link between HIV infection and AIDS in the face of overwhelming evidence provided by the global scientific community… [T]he president, the minister of health, and others in the government have long publicly denied the link between HIV and AIDS…

Though the media have asserted this innumerable times, there is interestingly no basis for it. Mbeki never denied the link between HIV and AIDS, as I will show in Chapter Three.

But more than this, the footnote Benatar uses to support his contention actually opens a door to some of the deeper issues of why we have trouble hearing black African voices. To Benatar, the important question was not Mbeki's contribution, but whether or not the dissident scientists were correct, and the footnoted article by the president of the South African Medical Research Council, MW Makgoba, indeed roundly criticized the dissidents.[7] However, Makgoba had far more to say in that article.

He began with a summary of what the current South African government "under President Thabo Mbeki" had done regarding AIDS, concluding that its "preventive and management programs are the envy of the world," and lauding the "spirit of scientific independence within the broader framework of the African context, consciousness, conscience and social responsibility." Then, after his critique of the dissident scientists, he asked, "why do the media of our country fail to highlight these positive initiatives and report accurately on the nature of this controversy?" He went on, "the media has also failed to see the big picture – the picture of an international holistic strategy that links the whole HIV/AIDS epidemic to national socio-economic and national development. The emphasis here is about solutions rather than causation." By highlighting "this holistic approach", which he attributed to the UN and other international agencies, he was pointing beyond simply settling the microbial etiology question. Having already declared his allegiance to the HIV-causes-AIDS position, his critique of the media was for being stuck on the dissident question, reporting it inaccurately, and failing to report the positive activities of the South African government. None of this made it to the *New England Journal of Medicine* article. Why?

Let's step back a minute and look at the elements of this story. The conventional perception is that Mbeki communicated with dissidents, therefore Mbeki was a dissident, therefore he should be exposed and countered. This view exists because the mainstream media – which saw some of Mbeki's speeches and interviews as ambiguous – presented it this way. (We will look at these speeches and interviews in Chapter Three). Makgoba, as we saw, felt that the media failed to report accurately.

In addition, Mbeki's approach was not limited to the biomedical model in his analysis of AIDS, an approach he shared with Treichler and the authors of *Beyond Epidemiology*, as we saw above. However, the biomedical model remains dominant in the West. Scholars who quietly depart from it are tolerated; well-known politicians who depart from it and may be able to influence policy are not.

Taken together, then, we have a well-known politician who departs from narrow biomedical scientific hegemony and is reported inaccurately by the media. The extent of the emotional response to this, the hostility, the consensus that Mbeki was wrong, and the disproportionate estimate of the danger of Mbeki's stance, all suggest that the public reaction to Mbeki was a "moral panic" – part of what we used to call crowd psychology. Examples in the West might be public reaction to marijuana use or flag burning.

Two sociologists, Erich Goode and Nachman Ben-Yehuda, describe moral panics as episodes when "people have become intensely concerned about a particular issue or perceived threat – which, as measured by concrete indicators, turns out to be not especially damaging – and have assembled, and taken action, to remedy the problem; yet, somehow, at a later point in time, they lost interest in the issue or threat, often turning their attention to other matters."[8]

Activists often drive moral panics, so their activity in the Mbeki story is no surprise. What makes this moral panic particularly interesting is that liberal activists, who in other situations might be among the first to advocate for African voices, have been in the forefront of the critique of Mbeki. This has been true both within South Africa (the Treatment Action Campaign mentioned in *Beyond Epidemiology*) as well as in the West. There are at least two reasons for this. First, the most recent generation of African leaders – the "Big Men" like Mobutu, Moi, Banda, Amin, Bokassa, Houphouët-Boigny, and so on – have been autocratic and have enriched themselves from their nation's wealth. Activists would naturally be suspicious of those in power in Africa.

The second reason is more subtle. Activists, in deciding what to advocate for, are often rooted in a particular religious or political paradigm. For health activists, that paradigm is usually the biomedical paradigm which has been so successful in creating responses to disease – the same biomedical paradigm shared by the society at large. These activists don't question those medical responses, they simply advocate that they be shared equally rather than be available only to the rich. Mbeki, while not opposed to the biomedical paradigm, did not think it was the only way to understand AIDS in South Africa. In questioning some of the responses declared – demanded even – by that paradigm, Mbeki became the target of the activists rather than their ally.

One way, then, to understand the negative public reaction to Mbeki is to see the entire situation as a moral panic. While that may help to explain why "Mbeki's more insightful statements on poverty's role in creating AIDS in the South African context" have been "silenced", it can only help explain an event, not a chronic situation. It still does not explain why the writers of *Beyond Hunger in Africa* felt excluded. Why, then, is it so difficult for the West to hear African voices like these?

The underlying questions here are questions of knowledge and power – questions openly debated in the academic world, but often invisible to the public. What is True, how we decide what's True – and who decides – are critical questions, but can seem obscure and arcane even to a concerned and literate public, and especially the

17

part of that public who lean toward activism rather than philosophy. The discussions are, nonetheless, important. Let us listen to what two Africans say about why we have trouble hearing them; the first relates to power, the second to knowledge.

> "With AIDS we are seeing a replay of a dynamic which has occurred between the Third World, particularly Africa, and the West many times before," says Nigerian Eddie Iroh, a senior international journalist [who was at the time European editor of the *African Guardian* magazine.]
> "The Western media is bigger and better funded, and possesses superior communication technology, than the Third World, and so its voice is most often heard. This dominance makes it difficult for Africans to air their points of view, and especially to combat what many see as anti-African propaganda."[9]

The point here is not whether or not the media is reporting accurately, but which media is doing the reporting. It is difficult to hear African voices simply because they are not as loud as the Western ones.

But, we may respond, facts are facts, regardless of who reports them. Yet even that defense carries an assumption: that there is such a thing as a culture-free fact, and that the methods of science are value-free. More and more voices are saying they are not. V. Y. Mudimbe, an African philosopher, commenting on how Westerners have viewed him and his continent, describes the Western "epistemological ethnocentrism; namely, the belief that scientifically there is nothing to be learned from 'them' unless it is already 'ours' or 'us.'"[10] His simple and subtle sentence contains a profound point: how people from the West listen to voices from Africa is predetermined by what they already know. Our Western scientific paradigm inhibits us from hearing the knowledge born in other paradigms. But more than this, Mudimbe is suggesting that it is very difficult for people in the West to hear *anything* from Africa. In other words, it is difficult for the West to hear African voices because, to us, *there are no African voices* different from our own voice. The ultimate fate of epistemological ethnocentrism, or epistemological arrogance, is to be alone, unencumbered and unaffected by other views, isolated from them so much that we don't realize they exist.

But they do exist. There are African voices, different from the voices that won't stop talking long enough to realize that there are other voices. Our first step must be to stop talking. And then listen, listen carefully.

References

[1] **Bond, GC et al (1997):** *AIDS in Africa and the Caribbean* (Boulder, Colorado, Westview Press,), p. xiii.

[2] **Achebe, C, Hyden, G, Magadza, C, and Okeyo, AP (1990):** *Beyond Hunger in Africa: Conventional Wisdom and an African Vision,* (Nairobi, Heinemann).

[3] **Achebe, C et al,** *Ibid,* **1990.**

[4] **Treichler, Paula (1999):** *How to Have Theory in an Epidemic: Cultural Chronicles of AIDS* (Durham, North Carolina, Duke University Press), p. 99, 125.

[5] **Kalipeni, E, Craddock, S, Oppong, J, and Ghosh, J (2004):** *HIV and AIDS in Africa: Beyond Epidemiology,* (Malden, Massachusetts, Blackwell Publishing), p. 4-5.

[6] **Benatar, Solomon (2004):** "Health Care Reform and the Crisis of HIV and AIDS in South Africa," *NEJM* 351:1 p. 81-92.

[7] **Makgoba, MW (2002):** "Politics, the media and science in HIV/AIDS: the peril of pseudoscience," *Vaccine* 20, p. 1899-1904.

[8] **Goode, E and Ben-Yehuda (1994):** N, *Moral Panics: The Social Construction of Deviance* (Cambridge, Massachusetts, Blackwell), p. 4, 33-41.

---

[9] Quoted in **Renee Sabatier (ed.) (1988):** *Blaming Others: Prejudice, Race, and Worldwide AIDS* edited by Renee Sabatier (Washington DC, New Society Publishers), the Panos Institute Report p. 97-98.

[10] **Mudimbe, VY (1988):** *The Invention of Africa: Gnosis, Philosophy, and the Order of Knowledge* (Bloomington, Indiana, Indiana University Press) p. 15.

1

"Are We Satisfied...?":
Seeking Distinctly African Views

Kenneth Kaunda has excellent AIDS-fighting credentials. He was the first reigning African president to openly admit there was AIDS in his family. After he was voted out of office in Zambia—a defeat he accepted non-violently—he set up a foundation for the care of African children with AIDS. When George Bush signed his $15 billion AIDS bill for Africa on May 27, 2003, Kenneth Kaunda was in the audience. Bush had this to say about Kaunda:

> It is my honor to recognize Dr. Kenneth Kaunda, the former President of Zambia... We see hope in the work of individuals like the former President of Zambia who lost his son to AIDS, a son who left several children to the care of their grandfather. The good President turned his grief to good works and created the Kenneth Kaunda Children of Africa Foundation. His foundation pays for food and medical care and schooling for AIDS orphans. Mr. President, we honor you for your service and for the example you have shown to others who live on your ravished continent. Thank you for coming today, sir. (Applause.) ...[1]

I had an appointment to interview former President Kaunda the week before in Boston, where he was on an assignment for Boston University, and I was in town for my daughter Elizabeth's graduation from the same university. Kaunda postponed the interview because he was attending Walter Sisulu's funeral in South Africa. As I had to leave Boston on the same day Bush was praising Kaunda, Elizabeth, who had set up the interview, was left to conduct it without me.

21

On June 2, during the interview, she asked him if he agreed with Mbeki that the root of the problem of AIDS was poverty. He answered:

> Can we look at it from any other angle? Do we understand the problem of AIDS? Certainly not. Why do I say so? Here in Europe-America-Western countries, where the cost, the standard of living is high, you fight HIV-AIDS very effectively, because people live on $1200, $12000... am I right? a year, and we live on $100. Ok? If you're lucky.... If we improve the standard of living in Africa tomorrow, you improve the life too. Even though you are sick, you are stronger... I have seen... a man in the World Bank, HIV positive, and he is strong! Naturally strong. And it is because he is eating properly, bathing properly, doing everything properly. Because he has the means to. So, I think that comment has been deliberately misunderstood—I shouldn't say deliberately, I withdraw "deliberately"—has been misunderstood.[2]

Kaunda's diplomatic defense of Mbeki is far from unusual. The most striking anomaly of the Mbeki AIDS story, which we will consider in Chapter 3, is not how the Western media misrepresented him, but rather how different the Western response to him was from the African response. Kaunda softened his critique of the media, but he did not soften his defense of Mbeki.

The first time I realized that there was a specifically African view of AIDS—or even that there was more than one way to see the disease—was in mid 2000. I was living in Kenya, working in a hospital where "treating AIDS" meant only treating the infections that result when a person's immunity is lowered. I discovered a pamphlet produced by a consortium of Kenyan AIDS organizations, and in their June 2000 edition the editor, Oyunga Pala, said that there had emerged in Africa a "loose confederacy of what some have termed as 'AIDS dissidents'" who "agree on one umbrella question: Are we satisfied—or to what extent are we satisfied — with the answers which the scientific establishment has offered regarding HIV/AIDS medical theory and development?"[3]

The context was the growing dispute in the media surrounding Mbeki's views on AIDS, and especially his inviting some scientific "dissidents" to sit on his panel with "orthodox" scientists and discuss approaches to AIDS in Africa. Pala, known mostly for his columns about contemporary romance and relationships in the Saturday magazine section of the *Daily Nation* newspaper, had articulated in one brief non-threatening sentence the essence of the problem.

In some ways, Pala's question was no different from the questions that gay activists in the US had been asking of the medical establishment for nearly two decades. In fact, a similar question had been articulated academically in an article published in the *American Journal of Public Health* seven years earlier[4] — as well as in several books such as those mentioned in the Prologue of this book. But, as was stated in the *AJPH* article, in the paradigm of biomedical individualism "only scientists and physicians are seen as possessing the expertise to define disease and frame research questions," not presidents. Gay men were angry enough, organized enough, and articulate enough to finally be heard by the scientific establishment. Mbeki was one man, crucified by the Western media, and not taken seriously by scientists and physicians.

Yet for many African scholars, Mbeki's views on AIDS struck a chord they resonated with; Mbeki became for them the starting point of their own reflections. Pala's question introduced me to a discourse of AIDS in Africa far broader than the merely biomedical. It showed me that while the "dissident" discourse is the minority view of the West, it is the foundational view of Africans — if we understand that Pala's broader view of "dissident" does not refer primarily to dissent from scientific "facts", but rather to satisfaction with scientific answers. Seeing how Mbeki was interpreted across the continent suggests that far from being a dissident in the 'denialist' sense, he was the spokesperson for a widely held view of AIDS far more inclusive than the narrow biomedical view that has hegemony in the West.

Initially, at least, he was the spokesperson. But political realities in South Africa pushed him to back off from this role in 2002. By then it was clear that he was no longer *the* spokesperson for an African view, but rather a catalyst for African *views*. This book concerns how these views developed.

In order to understand the development of the African AIDS discourses catalyzed or echoed by Mbeki, we must first sketch the intellectual background and explain some terms. A *discourse* is a conversation. The root word for discourse means "to run to and fro" - a conversation goes back and forth between participants who have something in common with each other. What they have in common determines the assumptions, the content, and the boundaries of the conversation. Because discourses are limited in this way, no single discourse can exhaust a topic.

Clearly the dominant discourse about AIDS today—at least for the media and the public—is the biomedical discourse. This is the point of view that considers AIDS mainly as an infectious disease, caused by a virus called HIV, usually transmitted sexually or by blood contact. In this conversation, prevention means keeping the virus away from people by using clean needles, safe blood products, and especially "safe sex": condoms or abstinence. Treatment means treating the infections that result from a lowered immunity, and increasingly it means using complicated expensive drug regimens to inhibit the growth of the virus itself. This is the conversation that is at the core of most international AIDS conferences. Because it is primarily scientific and technical, the centers of research for this discourse are in the West and the participants, while truly international, conduct their discussion in these Western terms.

There are of course many other conversations taking place around the world about AIDS. For example, a tiny dissident discourse dissents from the scientific majority and denies that HIV causes AIDS. However, most discourses do not take issue with the "facts" of the biomedical discourse, but simply emphasize the contexts in which AIDS exists: cultural, social, economic, political, philosophical, theological, gender, etc. Because these conversations see the importance of the cultural or economic or political settings, they may raise questions about the application of the biomedical approaches—or, as Pala said, "the answers which the scientific establishment has offered." Consequently, any discourse other than the biomedical can appear to be "dissident", even though it does not question the "facts" of science.

Now, since about two-thirds of the world's AIDS burden is supposedly in Africa, it is clear that we must try to understand how Africans understand their own epidemic; that is, what the African discourses are. This can be more difficult than it seems. In the same way that the biomedical discourse overshadows all other AIDS discourses, so the Western discourses, both biomedical and non-biomedical, can overshadow the African discourses. Yet, says Professor Jesse Mugambi of Nairobi University, in seeking to understand African discourses, "it is not and it will never be possible for a foreigner to understand Africans entirely... Interpreting African life using foreign norms as the criteria... will distort the real nature of African life... The ideal [in research] would be to have Africans who are academically disciplined and who at the same time remain full participants in their ethnic communal life."[5] It is important, in other words, to listen to and work with African scholars trained and working in Africa.

We can see the need to listen to African scholars *living and working in Africa* by looking at the views of Dr. Chinua Akukwe. Dr. Akukwe is an African professor of public health at George Washington University who has lived in the US for many years. He is also former vice chairman of the National Council for International Health (now renamed the Global Health Council), and is on the board of directors of the Constituency for Africa, an American advocacy coalition for Africa rooted in the African-American community. He is, in other words, well-respected in the West. Akukwe has written extensively about AIDS in Africa, especially since the International AIDS meeting in Durban in 2000. We will consider some of what he has written, not because his views are unique, but because they highlight the difference between "standard" Western understandings articulated by Africans living in the West, and the discourse as it is developing in Africa.

Professor Akukwe's view of the African AIDS epidemic is clearly rooted in his public health orientation, an orientation that accepts the biomedical approach to the disease, and tries to apply it to large populations. His approach in most articles is to begin with a review of the statistics about AIDS in Africa, followed by a listing of some problems the disease causes in Africa, and concluding with a list of suggestions.

Several themes recur. His statistics are usually dramatic and foreboding, his predictions dire. "The HIV/AIDS crisis in Africa is the most devastating disaster to befall the continent," he says. "Within the last two decades, the AIDS virus is responsible for ten times more deaths in Africa than all wars combined."[6] "There is even the ominous possibility nation-states in Africa may implode from the unprecedented assault of AIDS. In 16 countries, 1 in 10 adults live with the virus. For some countries, the toll is mind boggling: Botswana, 1 in 3 adults; Zambia, 1 in 4; South Africa, 1 in 5. Hardest-hit countries face the prospect of losing 25 percent of their productive citizens to AIDS within the next decade."[7]

Then, in reviewing the problems caused by AIDS, and the problems Africa has in confronting the epidemic, his observations are not surprising: AIDS flourishes where there is poverty, AIDS causes more poverty, and the poverty of African governments and their health care infrastructure make it even more difficult for them to confront and control the epidemic.

His suggestions are manifold, but in most articles include the following elements:

1. Responses must be African. "Africa must stop looking outside the continent for leadership in the fight against HIV/AIDS."[8] "No external agency will do for Africa what Africans must do for themselves."[9] "The ultimate responsibility for managing and eventually conquering the HIV/AIDS menace lie with Africans, in the continent and the Diaspora."[10]

2. As just noted, the African Diaspora has a special responsibility to be involved.

3. The response must include anti-retroviral drugs. "For quite sometime, some experts considered it 'irrational,' 'impractical,' or 'sheer fantasy' to talk about the need for the international

community to provide life saving drugs to AIDS patients in the hardest-hit countries. Now, the argument is shifting to 'When, Where, and How,' the international community can deliver lifesaving drugs to all AIDS patients, especially in Africa."[11] "The medical and health related aspects of HIV/AIDS include a strong resolution to provide life-saving drugs to Africans living with HIV/AIDS."[12] "The African Union meetings for this year should quickly take a stand and initiate action on access to lifesaving medicines for the nearly 30 million people living with AIDS on the continent."[13]

4. The international community, and especially the United States, needs to be more involved, especially by advocating for cheaper medicines and debt relief for African countries.

5. Africa needs to change. "Without dictating their actions, the US should work with African governments to ensure movement in the following areas: (a) allocation of more money by African nations to fight AIDS; (b) sustained political reforms to encourage pluralistic political and multi-sectoral campaigns against AIDS; (c) end corrupt practices that siphon foreign aid and investments; and (d) encourage the emergence of more civil society involvement in politics and non-government programs at community levels."[14] And, "African governments should become enablers of private enterprises."[15]

At first glance, none of this is surprising, nothing that he said is "wrong". This description and these prescriptions for AIDS in Africa mirror the conventional public health wisdom of the West— with the added advantage that the author has more credibility because he is an African. In fact, he emphasizes this identity in the title of his article published in South Africa's *Business Day* on May 21, 2001: "AIDS: An African Response". Akukwe clearly represents an African discourse on AIDS, one that many African professionals both on the continent and in the Diaspora undoubtedly subscribe to. That it mirrors the biomedical and public health discourses of the West—that it is *not* dissident—does not make it any less African, or at least any less Africanist.

However, there are a few clues in Akukwe's writing that suggest he may not have his ear to the ground with respect to broader grassroots African opinion and African scholarship. In an early article written with Melvin Foote about the Durban AIDS conference in 2000, they said, "A popular African government tasted the raw anger of its citizens. The harsh criticism that reportedly heralded the keynote speech of the host head of state, President Mbeki, during the Conference and swift, widespread bitterness regarding the perceived lack of action by the South African government on HIV/AIDS, should serve as a wake up call to African governments."[16] Shortly before this, Akukwe ended another article on the conference with this veiled reference to Mbeki: "The time to act is now to save lives and create a better future for Africa. The much vaunted African renaissance will become a pipedream if African intellectuals and leaders waste time chasing shadows while the proverbial Rome burns. The die is cast."[17] A year later he said, "President Thabo Mbeki is yet to publicly retreat from his intellectual excursions delinking AIDS from HIV."[18]

From the beginning, Akukwe took sides with the activists in South Africa and the Western press, and consequently against the widespread but quieter support for Mbeki throughout the rest of Africa. He has developed a thorough and reasonable analysis of AIDS in Africa, rooted in the Western public health discourse—but there is little that is *distinctively* African about his approach. He is, to quote Pala, "satisfied... with the answers which the scientific establishment has offered regarding HIV/AIDS medical theory and development." He apparently sees no need to listen to African scholars trained and working in Africa; the "facts" of the epidemic are clear. What is needed is "less talk and more action"—the title of his July 24, 2000 article.

What this analysis of Akukwe illustrates is that the way we understand anything involves assumptions, and that often these assumptions—including the entire agenda and the "terms of debate"—are set in the West. We don't listen to Africans in Africa because it doesn't occur to us that they may have a different way of looking at things, as we suggested in the Prologue. Dr. Laurenti Magesa, writing about "The Expatriate Worker in Africa", says:

> For real or imagined reasons, some of 19th century
> derogatory descriptions of Africa by Western
> organizations are returning with force, and with them
> similar attitudes. The real reasons are the increase in inter-
> ethnic violence, famine, and the spread of AIDS in Africa.
> The imagined reasons, which are much more responsible
> for shaping Western attitudes, are the belief that the
> extermination of the African peoples is imminent on
> account of these calamities. Without the intervention of the
> West, it is thought, Africa is doomed.
>
> So Western organizations — religious, governmental and
> nongovernmental — are pouring into Africa. They come
> bearing all sorts of unsolicited gifts and advice. The advice
> ranges from how to plant trees to how to get married, and
> even how to bury the dead! You can fill in anything in
> between. Much of this advice consists of answers to
> unasked questions.[19]

AIDS is one reason the West pays attention to Africa, but that attention is in the form of rescuing, not learning. The West doesn't seem to realize that there are African discourses of AIDS fundamentally different from the Western discourses, but the debate over Mbeki's views on AIDS has brought this difference to the surface. These discourses are not merely the quiet journalistic voices that defended Mbeki in 2000-2002. These are scholarly African analyses — but they are mostly hidden precisely because they are taking place in Africa, and the "terms of debate" have not yet included a serious recognition that there are other ways to see the epidemic, especially if those ways appear to be "dissident".

We must listen to the African discourses. There are already too many "white elephants" in Africa, too many development projects that have missed the mark. The AIDS problem is not the place to once again introduce inappropriate Western responses, and then blame Africa — or just slink away — when those responses fail. We must find and understand and listen to the African discourses. Though it is still too early to see them in perspective, I would like to tell six representative stories of how the African discourses are developing.

We will begin by reviewing the coverage of AIDS over the last decade in a magazine published by and for Africans, the *New African*. While it is not an academic journal, and the writing seems sometimes sensational to Western readers, the articles often reflect the questions in the minds of many Africans. These questions provide the beginnings of the African discourse of AIDS.

Following this, we will look carefully at the events surrounding South African President Thabo Mbeki's views on AIDS, especially in 2000-2001. The story needs to be revisited: many Westerners know Mbeki only because of press reports on his views on AIDS, leading them to think he is a crazy despot. Others who know more about him are confused about how such an intelligent respectable leader could have such strange views—strange, at least, to Westerners. There is a need to set the record straight, at least; to consider what Mbeki actually said, to suggest alternative explanations than those of the mainstream press, and to see how other African scholars view him.

The third story is about a particular conference held in Uganda in response to the negative Western press about Mbeki, and is worth considering in detail. Though the conference was organized by Western "dissidents", there were several papers presented by African scholars, papers that went beyond the fruitless debates about the origins of AIDS, or the unhelpful debates about whether or not the virus had been isolated. At this conference, a mature African discourse on AIDS—different from the "dissident" discourse, but also different from the mainstream—began to be articulated.

Meanwhile, African scholars had been quietly contributing to the mainstream discourses in theology and the social sciences, and a careful look at some of these articles reveals some distinctive African analyses. We will first look at African philosophy and theology as foundations of the way Africans have developed their perspectives on AIDS. We will then consider some African writings on gender issues, gender being a pivotal focus in contemporary African thinking on AIDS.

Returning to the public arena, we will use an international AIDS conference held in Nairobi in 2003 as a case study of how the African news media covered this event. This conference occurred about the same time as President George Bush announced a major plan for the US to confront African AIDS, mostly by paying for antiretroviral drugs, and this announcement provided the backdrop for the African press coverage of the conference.

Finally, African artists have not surprisingly been wrestling with their epidemic, in media ranging from theater and music to the plastic arts. Although books are not as plentiful in Africa as in the West, fiction writers as well have been reflecting on the AIDS epidemic in the stories they write. In the concluding chapter we will look at a dozen novels published in eastern and southern Africa, all written by Africans. While never claiming to be "programs" to control AIDS, they still reflect the questions in the minds of many Africans—bringing us back to the subject of the first story. It is crucial to be aware of these questions: as the Western discourse develops in response to Western questions, so the African discourse has been developing in response to African questions. As a postscript, we will look briefly at mourning. Africa, beset by too much dying from AIDS, mourns. Is there a way we can join Africa in this mourning? Can mourning lead us to understand more fully how Africa feels about AIDS, and how we might be able to help?

References

---

[1] *http://www.whitehouse.gov/news/releases/2003/05/20030527-7.html*

[2] **Kenneth Kaunda (2003),** interviewed by Elizabeth Downing, Boston, MA, June 2, 2003.

[3] **Oyunga Pala (2000),** "A word from the editor," *Partner: The Newsletter of the Kenyan AIDS NGOs Consortium,* June, 2000, p.2.

[4] **Fee, Elizabeth and Krieger, Nancy (1993),** "Understanding AIDS: Historical Interpretations and the Limits of Biomedical Individualism," *American Journal of Public Health,* Oct. 1993, vol 83, no 10, p. 1477-1486.

[5] **Mugambi, J.N.K (1989),** *Christianity and African Culture* (Acton Publishers, Nairobi), p.188-9.

[6] **Akukwe, Chinua (2000a),** "HIV/AIDS in Africa: Less Talk and More Action," July 24, 2000, in *www.afbis.com/analysis/aids.htm*

[7] **Akukwe, Chinua (2000b),** "Africa's HIV/AIDS dilemma," *The Washington Times,* Nov 26, 2000.

[8] **Akukwe, Chinua (2003),** "HV/AIDS and Africa: Back to the Drawing Board," *Addis Tribune* (Ethiopia), January 10, 2003.

[9] **Akukwe, Chinua (2001),** "AIDS: An African Response," *Business Day* (South Africa), May 21, 2001.

[10] **Akukwe,** *op. cit.,* **2000a.**

[11] **Foote, Melvin, and Akukwe, Chinua (2000),** "HIV/AIDS in Africa: The Gains of the Durban Conference," September 9, 2000, in *www.afbis.com/analysis/hiv.htm.*

[12] **Akukwe,** *op. cit.,* **2003.**

[13] **Akukwe, Chinua,** "HIV/AIDS, Africa and 2003: Urgent Strategic Issues," in *http://chora.virtualave.net/akukwe-hiv2.htm.*

[14] **Akukwe, Chinua and Foote, Melvin (2001),** "HIV/AIDS in Africa: Time to Stop the Killing Fields", April 2001, in *www.fpif.org/briefs/vol6/v6n15hivafrica_body.html.*

[15] **Akukwe,** *op. cit.,* **2001.**

[16] **Foote and Akukwe,** *op. cit.,* **2000.**

[17] **Akukwe,** *op. cit.,* **2000a.**

[18] **Akukwe,** *op. cit.,* **2001.**

[19] **Magesa, Laurenti (2002),** *Christian Ethics in Africa,* (Nairobi, Acton Publishers), p. 112-113.

2

The *New African*:
The Beginnings Of An African Discourse On AIDS

Introduction

Almost every busy street corner in downtown Nairobi has them: the magazine sellers. They have piles of three or four newspapers and more than a dozen colorful glossy magazines spread out in front of them on the sidewalk, each pile with a rock or piece of thick beveled glass keeping it from blowing away. There are the local variants of *True Confessions* (the cover may be glossy, but there is newsprint inside), sometimes the *National Geographic*, and several economic and political news magazines. Prominent among them is the *New African* magazine, which calls itself "the oldest pan-African monthly in English". Based in London, with a continent-wide circulation of 32,000, this glossy magazine often has a close-up photograph of a prominent African on the cover, a promise of an "untold story" or a special report inside, and articles with titles that often end in question marks. The magazine wants you to buy it, and promises you a cutting-edge, questioning analysis when you do.

Not surprisingly, the *New African* has been covering news and viewpoints about African AIDS over the last decade—and, in line with their desire to tell a different "inside" story, their coverage has not followed the Western "orthodox" line. In other words, their coverage has been controversial. Though they never received as much media attention as Mbeki would several years later, their coverage in the 90s was different enough from the conventional story to merit two articles in the Western press—and both missed the point.

The first was released by the Knight Ridder/Tribune News Service on Aug 12, 1999, and appeared in several US papers in the next few days. The author was Neely Tucker, a white Zimbabwean journalist, and the subject matter was how the *New African* had been covering AIDS—or more accurately, how badly they had been covering it. The *San Diego Union Tribune* titled their article "AIDS Just a Sinister Hoax, Many Africans Told: Intellectuals Spread Message of Denial"; the title of the original story from the News Service was only slightly less inflammatory: "AIDS Workers Say Denial, Paralyzing Fatalism Are Biggest Obstacles". Neely interviewed the editor, Baffour Ankomah, reviewed some of the *New African* articles, and concluded that Ankomah "wants to convince his readers that there is no such thing as AIDS and that millions of Africans aren't dying of it.... The magazine's editorials urge people to ignore health warnings and to not wear condoms."[1]

Six months later, a dissident website called Rethinking AIDS published their opinion of *New African*'s AIDS coverage in an article titled "Major African Magazine Reappraises HIV-AIDS Model." It said: "Led by Baffour Ankomah, *New African* scrutinizes reports of doomsday epidemic and assumption that HIV is the cause." This article praised *New African*'s dissenting views, focusing especially on coverage of those who question the viral cause of AIDS. *New African* dispatches, said the article, "accurately consider the conclusions of Duesberg, Eleopulos, and others who propose non-HIV explanations for AIDS.... Mostly, though, *New African* stories stress the views of Duesberg and (increasingly) Eleopulos."[2]

Both articles, it's true, gave more extensive analysis than these few sentences early on in each article. Both commented on *New African*'s questioning of official statistics about the extent of the epidemic, both mentioned that *New African* had been questioning conventional wisdom about the origin of AIDS, both commented on the difficulty of using clinical diagnosis as a basis for statistics. All these issues, as we will see, were central in the *New African* coverage. But each article began with what was most important to the author: whether or not HIV causes AIDS. The Neely article criticized *New African* for not believing that HIV was the cause; the Rethinking AIDS article praised them for exactly the same reason.

In fact, the viral cause of AIDS has never been the chief concern of the *New African*, one way or the other. "Ankomah declines to endorse or reject any of the major explanations of AIDS, including the HIV model. 'I am not an expert,' he told *RA*. 'I don't know what causes AIDS, if HIV is harmless, if it causes AIDS, or if it's merely an artifact.'"[3]

This not knowing is very difficult for Westerners to handle, especially when a journalist writing about AIDS claims not to know. For Westerners, both orthodox and dissident, this is the starting point—and the end point. When Mbeki raised questions about conventional wisdom of AIDS, as we will see, the scientific response to him was not to deal with his questions, but to *declare* in the Durban Declaration that HIV was the cause of AIDS. If someone questions that viral cause, the assumption is also that they reject standard health warnings, as Neely assumed. Ankomah answered him this way: "As our worldwide readers are well aware, never ever has *New African* written editorials 'urging people to ignore health warnings and not to wear condoms.' This is purely a figment of Neely's imagination. Bad propaganda, I hasten to add."[4]

Likewise for dissidents, when someone expresses doubts about the orthodox position, that person is celebrated, as the extensive coverage of Mbeki by dissident websites shows—even if microbial cause is not their concern, as it wasn't with Ankomah. Apparently some Africans don't think that having a detailed understanding of the microscopic cause is necessary in order to analyze and approach the macroscopic epidemic. Despite the claim of Rethinking AIDS, neither the views of Duesberg nor those of Eleopulos are at that center of the *New African* analysis.

If the *New African* is neither orthodox nor dissident, what then is it? The reality is that Western analysts do not have a category for what the *New African* is doing. Its approach has been mostly to raise questions and expose alternative points of view, but the result may be the beginnings of an authentically African discourse on AIDS

Overview

The beginnings of an African discourse on AIDS, at least in the *New African*, were clearly with the Western dissidents. Over half of the authors writing about AIDS in the magazine in the mid-90s were not African; most of these were Western dissidents. In 1994, Dr. Charles Geshekter, the dissident professor of African History, had an article; in 1996, it was Neville Hodgkinson, a dissident British journalist; in 1997, Dr. Rosalind Harrison, who with her husband Richard Chirimuuta had published *AIDS, Africa and Racism* in 1987; and in 1998 Christian Fiala, a dissident Austrian doctor whose focus is epidemiology.

What might be significant is who is missing from this list: Duesberg, Rasnick, Giraldo, and Eleopulos. All of these are scientists who dispute the HIV cause of AIDS, all were eventually on Mbeki's controversial AIDS Panel, and all have or are well represented on dissident websites. And, true enough, several are mentioned in Neville Hodgkinson's book *AIDS: The Failure of Contemporary Science* which was reviewed in the September 1996 issue of *New African*. However, the *New African* did not publish articles by these dissidents. Instead, they published articles questioning the origins of AIDS and statistical accuracy, articles like Geshekter's "Myths of AIDS and Sex" and Fiala's "Dirty Tricks Over AIDS Figures". It's not that the *New African* ignored the controversy over the viral cause; rather, they focused much more in the mid-90s on origins, statistics, and the accuracy of testing, as we shall see.

In June 1999 two events occurred which changed *New African's* coverage of AIDS. Baffour Ankomah, a Ghanaian, took over from Alan Rake, an Englishman, as editor of the magazine. And Mbeki became president of South Africa. Subsequently the number of articles on AIDS in *New African* greatly increased, fully three quarters of them were written by Africans, and almost every article contained a reference to Mbeki. And the themes they covered began to expand. *New African* still wrote about the inaccuracy of statistics and the AIDS tests, but they added coverage of anti-retroviral drugs and their toxicities, analysis of media coverage of

Mbeki, and the poverty which underlies the African AIDS epidemic. By 2003, when they published a speech on the politicization of AIDS by Dr. Peter Piot, the executive director of UNAIDS—clearly coming from an "orthodox" perspective—they had a firm African perspective for deciding which speech to publish.

Most of the more than 40 *New African* articles concerning AIDS published over the last decade dealt with one or more of the six themes just mentioned: origins of AIDS, accuracy of statistics, accuracy of testing, drug toxicities, media coverage (mostly in 2000), and poverty. We will examine each theme in detail, looking at some of the articles that expand on the theme, and begin to suggest how these themes lay a foundation for African discourses of AIDS.

To see these themes in perspective, it is interesting to look briefly at some other themes of African AIDS which the *New African* has dealt with only in passing, or not at all. The most prominent themes in the Western media have been the need for condoms, and more recently, the need for anti-retroviral drugs in Africa, both drawing heavily from the biomedical discourse. This discourse also uses statistics, as we saw with Dr. Akukwe—but more to frighten than to question. Then the social science discourses have brought in many other themes, such as stigma, gender, ethical issues, etc, which are important to those discussing them, but have received less attention in the media. The point here is not that the *New African* magazine "disagrees" with any of these themes; it has simply not dealt with them in much detail. Our task now is to examine in detail what the *New African* does think is important.

Origins

I found it interesting, working in East African hospitals in the mid-1990s, that people I talked to were very concerned with where AIDS came from. To me it was a moot point: AIDS existed, and our task was to treat it the best we could and try to prevent it. But for Africans I worked with, that wasn't enough. They wanted to

37

know—these rural people who had probably never read *New African*—if I really thought it originated in Africa. I didn't know, I didn't really care—and I didn't realize that I was being introduced to a key element of an African discourse of AIDS.

For the *New African*, at least three aspects of the origin question are important: African sexuality, viral origins in African primates, and HIV as a man-made weapon of biological warfare. We will look at some articles devoted to each.

In the October 1994 issue Charles Geshekter published an article entitled "Myths of AIDS and Sex"[5]. By the mid-1990s it was clear that the African AIDS epidemic was following a different pattern than that in the West. In North America and Europe, AIDS was still found primarily in men who had sex with men and in intravenous drug users, but in Africa the disease seemed to be transmitted primarily by heterosexual sex. Further, the epidemic was spreading much faster in Africa than in North America where it was first reported. Not everyone tried to explain this difference, but those who did often assumed that Africans were simply more promiscuous than Westerners.

That is the assumption that Geshekter, a professor of African History at California State University at Chico confronts: "In fact," he says, "there is little evidence to support Western perceptions of African sexual promiscuity." He discusses sexual behavior in several African cultures—behavior which was traditionally not promiscuous—and even cites a 1991 study of sexual activity in Uganda, revealing "behavior that was not very different from that of the West." Why then is AIDS so much more prevalent in Africa? Geshekter begins to suggest two reasons: either AIDS is not in fact as prevalent in Africa as it seems, or there are factors other than just sexual activity to account for its spread.

The possibility that AIDS may not be as prevalent as it seems is a theme *New African* would return to frequently. Before AIDS tests were readily available in Africa, the diagnosis was usually made clinically: seeing a combination of symptoms that were typical in AIDS patients. Unfortunately, these symptoms (cough, diarrhea, weight loss) were so common in other diseases that an individual presenting with them could simply have pneumonia and amoeba, not AIDS. Even when tests became available, there were many false positive results, especially due to conditions common in Africa — pregnancy, for example, or malaria. Consequently, when epidemiologists put together statistics for Africa, they based them on the only information they had, which included clinical guesses and false positive tests. Geshekter reminds us of all of this, and we will return to it.

The other possibility, that there are other factors to explain widespread immunodeficiency in Africa, is how Geshekter ends his article: "It is the political economy of underdevelopment, not sexual intercourse that is killing Africans... African poverty, not some extraordinary sexual behavior, is the best predictor of AIDS-defining diseases." Over five years later, Mbeki would make some of these same points.

The second origin question, that of a source of the HIV virus in African primates, is the subject of Baffour Ankomah's 1998 article "Monkey Business Over AIDS"[6]. The article was a commentary on the news suggesting that the original source of the AIDS virus was a central African chimpanzee. In the mid-1980s, the theory was that the AIDS virus came from the African green monkey, and somehow jumped to people. However, that theory had been abandoned: "the HIV virus and the monkey virus were so different from each other that none of them 'could have been the ancestor of the other in a historical past,'" wrote Baffour. He continued that a blood sample, taken from a man in Central Africa in 1959, had recently tested positive for HIV, and the Western press was reporting that this "proved" that AIDS started in Africa – probably in a chimpanzee from which viruses similar to AIDS had been found.

Much of Ankomah's article is a review of evidence that would cast doubt on this theory. He cites in detail work by other scientists which shows the unreliability of "positive" HIV tests in old frozen blood samples. He emphasizes that no one claims to know whether or not the 1959 man in central Africa was in fact African. And he quotes extensively from an article Dr. Rosalind Harrison wrote for the *New African* the year before. She had shown that there had been extensive contact between Africans and Europeans for over 400 years, giving plenty of opportunity for a virus that may have "jumped" from a primate to a human to spread to Europe—but that clearly did not happen.

The next article we will review picks up the same theme: "If chimps have been 'the natural host and reservoir for HIV-1... possibly dating to a period... several hundred thousand years ago,' why did HIV only infect humans ONLY in the 1980s in America? Why hasn't the virus wiped out Africa's population these 'several hundred thousand years'? And why do the chimps themselves not suffer from AIDS?"[7]

"So," Ankomah asks rhetorically in his article, "Africans began to have more sex in the 1950s?" But Geshekter had already shown in his article that this was more of a Western myth than an African reality. The theory of an African primate origin of AIDS was still only a theory—but it was one that Western researchers kept coming back to. Why? Ankomah quotes Dr Harrison again: "even 'normal' science does not function independently of its social, economic and political context... the political and economic priorities of government and industry now largely determine the allocation of funds. And, as scientists bring into their work their own particular cultural baggage, so too the results of their work are expected to conform with prevailing cultural norms or vested interests."

After this quote, Ankomah closes his article with a very revealing statement – revealing, at least, to Westerners who wonder why Africans are so concerned about origins: "In short, we can all go to sleep safely in our beds with the knowledge that the February announcement is another 'political' evidence being used to blame Africa for the origin of AIDS." Regardless of the intent of the researchers, whether "purely" scientific or heavily influenced by culture and politics, many Africans have interpreted the resulting findings as *blame*. Wrestling with origins must be a pivotal part of African discourses of AIDS.

"AIDS Originated in the U.S. Special Virus Program," declared the *New African* in April, 1999.[8] This third aspect of the origin of AIDS, that it was a virus developed by the U.S. military, is one that Ankomah had previously written about in a 1993 article, "The

American Connection" in which he speculated about a US biowarfare connection to AIDS.[9] The 1999 article (beginning with the emotion-laden question "Did AIDS really originate in Africa?"), also by Ankomah, is mostly about the story of the first chimpanzee that was found to have an AIDS-like virus. The chimp had been captured in Africa in 1959, but had lived most of her life in a US military research laboratory. When she died, her remains were sent to the National Cancer Institute at Fort Detrick, Maryland—the location of the Word War II era biowarfare program. Ankomah presents no evidence to substantiate his claim in the title of the article, but he does point out inconsistencies in the chimpanzee story.

A year and a half later, in a book review about the CIA's role in Lumumba's 1960 death in the Congo, Osei Boateng came back to the idea that the HIV virus may have been man-made[10]. He refers in passing to Edward Hooper's book *The River*, which suggests that HIV may have been inadvertently spread by live polio vaccine trials in Africa. His only problem with Hooper's thesis is that it doesn't go far enough. Hooper also assumes an African origin for HIV—that it originally came from African chimps, but may have contaminated polio virus grown in chimp kidneys. What Boateng finds troubling, and wants to question, is that HIV originated in Africa at all.

Neither Ankomah nor Boateng try to "prove" that HIV was created as an agent of bioterrorism. However, they do use what is known—the CIA's involvement in Africa, and the existence of a U.S. biowarfare program—to infer that a man-made origin is possible. Then, at the end of his article, Ankomah comes back to the question of blame, but this time in a larger context. He refers in his last sentence to "the AIDS establishment bent on blaming Africa for the origin of AIDS just to deflect the blame from the real culprits."

For people not used to considering African reactions to Western research, this questioning of origins may sound like paranoid conspiracy theories and nit-picking—or grasping at straws, hoping things aren't as bad as they seem. But for many Africans, the theories of African origins sound like blame—and in this context the offers of help from the West seem patronizing ("You got yourself in this mess, I'll help to pull you out"). The question of origin may not be the most important question in the African discourses, but it is the first. By the late 1990s, the *New African* had moved on to several other questions. It is good to remember that, for many Africans, the origin questions have still not been settled.

Testing

The next two issues we will consider that *New African* addressed are related: testing and statistics, because the statistics are often based on the results of tests. There were several articles beginning in 1998 devoted specifically to statistics, and we will eventually look at their claims. However, the prior question is the validity of the HIV tests, which the *New African* had been questioning since at least 1994. There were few articles devoted exclusively to testing, but over a dozen mentioned its inaccuracies. We will now look at a few of the references to see what the *New African* was concerned about.

In the 1994 Geshekter article discussed above, he claims thus: "HIV tests are notoriously unreliable in Africa. A 1994 study in the *Journal of Infectious Diseases* concluded that HIV tests were useless in central Africa, where the microbes responsible for tuberculosis, malaria, and leprosy were so prevalent that they registered over 70 percent false positive results."[11] Even "pregnancy itself can cause unknown numbers of non-specific results."[12] Eight years later the *New African* was still concerned: "In the developed world HIV testing consists of the Enzyme-Linked Immuno-Sorbent Assay (ELISA) test followed by the Western Blot test. This is because studies have shown that the ELISA test alone produces at least an 83% false positive test result rate. However, in Africa, due to lack of resources, testing usually consists of the ELISA test only."[13]

In addition, there is confusion about how the tests are interpreted. In December, 2002, *New African* published a portion of an ANC document which quoted Rian Malan's writing for the *Rolling Stone*. Malan was recounting a 1994 study done on 184 high-risk subjects in a South African mining camp. "Twenty-one of the subjects came up positive or borderline positive on at least one

ELISA. But the results were confusing. A locally manufactured test said 2 subjects were positive. A British test indicated 7, but different people in almost every case. A French test declared 14 were infected... Of the 21 subjects who tested positive, 16 had had recent malaria infections." So the researchers devised a method for absorbing malaria antibodies from the samples, "then re-tested them. 80% of the suspected HIV infections disappeared."[14]

The degree of inaccuracy noted here is remarkable—but of course *New African* is not a scientific journal; it is simply reporting what some authors found in the scientific literature. Undoubtedly people with a different bias would quote studies showing lower rates of false positivity. The point, though, is that any degree of inaccuracy is disturbing. There are at least two major reasons:

1) "As a diagnosis of HIV infection has such a profound effect on a person's life, it was considered of utmost importance that the tests are unimpeachably reliable."

2) "Since all epidemiological predictions concerning HIV/AIDS in South Africa [and most of Africa] are based on the results of such tests, their absolute reliability was declared to be of utmost importance."[15]

As a physician, I must constantly deal with the possibility of false positivity—with any laboratory test. The problem did not begin with HIV testing. "Absolute" and "unimpeachable" reliability are difficult to achieve. However, with a disease as widespread as AIDS, and with such devastating consequences for an individual with a positive test, it certainly is of "utmost importance" that the tests used in Africa be reliable—more reliable than they are now.

My own experience illustrates the concerns of the *New African*. In 1999, after a decade of working in East African hospitals where AIDS was common, my wife and I decided to get tested for HIV. We are both physicians, and statistics told us that one out of every 5 or 6 people we had operated on was HIV positive. Since we had stuck ourselves several times with needles while operating, and since we did not routinely test surgery patients for HIV, we knew there was a tiny but real chance that one of us could have been infected. The test we used was ELISA, the same one we used for all our patients. Mine came back negative; my wife's came back positive. I brought a second sample of her blood to a Nairobi hospital for confirmation by the Western Blot test; it came back "indeterminate".

This occurred just before our daughter's high school graduation and a trip to the US to get her started in college. It was a memorable, gut-wrenching trip. When we finally were able to get more complete blood work done in the US, we found that all her tests—Western Blot and viral load—were negative. My wife's positive test was simply and fortunately a false positive. How many Africans with diarrhea and cough "simply" have false positive HIV tests? What percentage of the frightening AIDS statistics were "fortunately" only based on false positives test results?

There is, however, one further point about testing. In June 2001 the *New African* published the transcript of a television interview with Mbeki about AIDS testing. The interviewer asked if Mbeki would take an HIV-AIDS test, and he responded that whether or not he took it was irrelevant. But, she asked, wouldn't it set an example? Mbeki responded:

> No, but it would be setting an example within the context of a particular paradigm.... Now I don't believe that stunts, publicity stunts, help in addressing the health needs of our people.... The Panel said one of the things we've got to do is to determine when you do an HIV test, what is the test testing. And those were the scientists: what is it measuring? So I go and do a test, I'm confirming a particular paradigm. It doesn't help in addressing this health need. Our focus must be how we do improve the health of our people, and that is what we are focused on.[16]

What did Mbeki mean by "confirming a particular paradigm"? He may have meant simply that if he took an AIDS test, he would be showing confidence in that test—whereas, as we have just seen, he had plenty of reason to doubt its accuracy. His response may have been simple common sense, resisting the assumption that a single blood test could tell him whether or not he was healthy. But in the context of the Presidential Panel whose report had just come out, he probably meant that taking a blood test would confirm his belief in the paradigm that HIV was the essence of AIDS; that it alone, without any co-factor such as poverty and its negative effects on health, was enough to cause an escalating AIDS epidemic. The question was not whether HIV caused AIDS or not; his administration had already declared that it assumed that HIV was causative. The question was whether HIV alone—for that is all the HIV test measured—was the cause.

Completely delinking HIV from AIDS may be fringe science, but talking of co-factors is not—and once again it was the *New African* which publicized this. Consider the following quote from an interview with Luc Montagnier, the co-discoverer of the HIV virus:

> At first, yes, we thought we had the best candidate for this virus to be the cause of AIDS. But after a while—even from the beginning actually—we thought maybe for the activation of that virus in cells, we had to, we need some co-factors. So I would agree that HIV by itself, or some strains of HIV are not sufficient to induce AIDS.[17]

It is now well accepted that the HIV virus is necessary, but sometimes not sufficient, to cause AIDS. For example, people with untreated sexually transmitted infections are much more likely to become infected with HIV than are people without those open sores – and people who are poor are less able to get treatment for those other infections. Are denialists those who reject HIV, or are they those who reject co-factors?

Statistics

During 1998-9, *New African* published their first three articles about AIDS statistics in Africa, and the titles tell their story: "Dirty Tricks Over AIDS Figures," "Are 26 Million Africans Dying of AIDS?" and "AIDS: Let Them Eat Their Figures". The first was written by a

European AIDS dissident; all other articles after that were by Africans. The essence of these articles was to question the accuracy of the statistics routinely used to describe African AIDS. In the first article, for example, Christian Fiala notes that WHO had been basing their statistics on the number of reported AIDS cases defined by a clinical definition of AIDS, not HIV blood tests. That would clearly be only an estimate. But since WHO knew that not all cases were being officially "registered", they used a multiplication factor to calculate an estimate. "In 1996, the WHO multiplied registered AIDS cases in Africa by 12. In 1997 this had jumped to 17." By the next year, the number of WHO reported cases was 47 times the registered cases.[18]

Baffour Ankomah continues in a similar vein, quoting from a UNAIDS document. After speaking of "recalculated current *estimates*... based on the previously published *estimates*," the document continues:

> Epimodel 2, a microcomputer program... was used to *calculate* the new estimates on prevalence and incidence of AIDS and AIDS deaths, as well as the number of children infected through mother-to-child transmission of HIV, taking into account age specific fertility *rates*. An additional spreadsheet model was used to *calculate* the number of children whose mothers had died of AIDS. *The current estimates do not claim to be an exact count of infections*... [italics mine].

Ankomah has serious doubts about the accuracy of these estimates: "The figures, therefore, do not reflect the true situation on the ground,"[19] he writes.

Four years later, the *New African* felt vindicated when the program manager of the Ghanaian National AIDS Control Programme, Dr. Kweku Yeboah, said: "No population-based study [on HIV and AIDS], which is based on blood samples, has ever been carried out in Ghana because of logistic and ethical constraints." The magazine continued: "For years, many people around the world, including President Thabo Mbeki of South

Africa and our own magazine, *New African*, have questioned how HIV and AIDS statistics on Africa are arrived at.... Now the Ghana experience of 'no blood-sample-based study ever done in the country' appears to threaten the whole credibility of those statistics."[20]

By December 2002, the matter was no clearer. In the ANC document that *New African* published, referred to above, there was a quote from a demographer who had been studying African mortality statistics. When asked about the high levels of HIV infection being reported, he said, "I don't have much faith. It's essentially a modeling exercise, and the exercise has always seemed to have a political dimension."[21]

The critique by *New African*, however, is not merely a dry debate about numbers. They had some very specific concerns about the apparent inaccuracies. First, several articles mentioned that the official statistics are usually quite alarming. Why would organizations publish such alarming statistics as "fact" when they are based only on estimates, computer modeling, and "calculations" rather than counting? "The only sense in such a form of presentation is that 'huge figures bring in large amounts of public money' into AIDS research and, by extension, into the pockets of the researchers."[22]

Second, Baffour Ankomah was concerned about the effect of these "alarming" statistics on attention given to other diseases, such as malaria. In 1998 he wrote, "Why, after the failures of the past decade in AIDS research and forecast, UNAIDS still wants the world to concentrate billions of dollars on HIV/AIDS—a 'disease' that is yet to be scientifically proven—at the expense of malaria, the already proven 'biggest killer' of Africans, should worry us all."[23]

While some readers may bristle at his questioning of the scientific basis for AIDS, his point about ignoring malaria is still worth considering. In an article chronicling a visit to Senegal to report on the "successes" there, he again showed that attention to AIDS—based on widely publicized statistics—"consigns malaria... to the back burner." "Prostitutes get free condoms (50 a week) supplied by some NGOs who in turn get their free supplies from USAID.... There is no NGO distributing free mosquito nets supplied free by USAID."[24] Even if AIDS has been scientifically proven, is that a reason to all but ignore another disease that kills a comparable number of Africans?

Finally, as we saw with the question of origins, there is the awkward matter of blame and its effects. Baffour Ankomah again: "Thus, for Africa's own self-belief and confidence, it is time African governments shed their apathy, spoke out and challenged these figures as the Haitians did in the early 1980s when they were falsely blamed for the origin of AIDS." Note: "for Africa's own self-belief and confidence." Ankomah is aware of how draining it is to always be considered "the worst." Commenting on the UN's liberal use of unproven statistics, "the most disturbing thing is that in their haste *to do Africa's image the most harm*, the UN agencies do not apparently cross-check with one another..." [emphasis mine].[25] And "when UNAIDS and WHO are putting their figures together, African voices are hardly heard."[26]

Another *New African* author, Muzondwa Banda, felt the same way. Commenting on a Zambian official questioning the "alarmist" UN statistics, Banda wrote, "...some African governments are not going to lie down and swallow any AIDS figures forced down their throats by the Western AIDS establishment."[27] The tone is unmistakable: estimates masquerading as statistics are dishonest, harmful, and just plain insulting.

Drugs

After Mbeki became President of South Africa and Baffour Ankomah became editor of *New African*, both in mid 1999, *New African* coverage of AIDS intensified. They continued to comment on the problems with testing and statistics, as we have seen, but began covering several other issues, mostly responding to the questions being raised by Mbeki and the negative attention he was getting in the media. Their first mention of Mbeki's contribution to the AIDS story was in December 1999 in an article titled "Mbeki's AIDS Bombshell"—and the article focused on Mbeki's concerns about the toxicity of the anti-AIDS drug AZT.[28]

All medicines have potential toxicities (doctors like to call them "side-effects"). Sometimes these negative effects are mild and rare, but with the stronger drugs used for the more serious medical conditions, the toxic effects can be quite common and severe. Doctors are willing to prescribe these drugs if they feel the benefits outweigh the risks of toxicity. Theoretically they inform patients of these risks and the decision is a joint one; practically, patients with severe, life-threatening illnesses often "choose" a drug that might save their life, even if using it involves new illnesses and pain. In the US, this whole process occurs in the context of drugs already approved by the Food and Drug Administration (FDA)—but of course their decision to approve, based on benefits and toxicities, must also be somewhat arbitrary.

The *New African's* contribution was not just to declare that AZT had toxicities, but to show how arbitrary the decision process could be. "Despite these shortcomings," the *New African* said, commenting on some trials exposing AZT's possible toxicities, "the drug was given a license. The concerns expressed by the people who knew about the shortcomings of the drug were thrown out the window following an intervention from the FDA, which was under both political and public pressure to fast-track the drug on the market." The usually cautious FDA apparently changed its rules because of political pressure from people who felt that drugs would be the answer to AIDS.

In May, 2000, the *New African* raised again one of the questions of "The Great AIDS Debate": "Is AZT more toxic than beneficial...?"[29] By September, reporting on the International AIDS conference in Durban, the *New African* showed more clearly the role of medicines and the companies that make them in how we debate and understand AIDS. "The big Western drug companies had made major contributions to the sponsorship of the conference and expected returns on their investments." But Mbeki challenged their hegemony:

> He had dared question the unquestionable: the inconclusive theory that Aids is solely caused by a virus called HIV. He had dared to threaten the very foundation

upon which is built a huge Aids edifice that feeds on the virus. Pharmaceutical companies, Aids researchers, the medical establishment, microbiologists, NGOs, entrepreneurs, you name it.... [T]he president, expected to make penance in front of the drug lords, was unyielding. He stuck to the cornerstone of his presidency which seeks to find African solutions to African problems, only too well aware that self-interest is the only guiding principle in the West's dealings with Africa.[30]

That last statement may be an opinion, but it is one with plenty of evidence to back it up—which the *New African* provided in their April 2001 issue. By this time, the pharmaceutical industry was in the news because of their lawsuit against the South African government—a lawsuit they eventually dropped. (The suit objected to a South African law which would allow the local manufacture of drugs which were still under patent in other countries.) Concurrent with this attention on the pharmaceutical industry, The *Guardian* newspaper in London published a series of articles in February, 2001 called "Dying for Drugs" in which they exposed the profit motive and self-interest of the big pharmaceutical companies. The *New African* felt this series was important enough to summarize in their article called "The Profits That Kill."[31] From ensuring that profits go to their home (Western) countries, to increasingly testing drugs in Third World countries—drugs that may only benefit the West—"The Profits That Kill" provided clear evidence that "self-interest is the only guiding principle in the West's dealings with Africa."

Media

New African may be part of the media, but it is certainly not part of the mainstream media. When that mainstream media criticized *New African's* coverage of AIDS, as we saw at the beginning of this chapter, the *New African* answered. In a-several-page article, Baffour Ankomah responded point by point to Neely Tucker's accusations, and gave his view of their interview.[32] Besides setting the record straight, the article also demonstrated how inaccurate the mainstream media could be.

New African returned to this theme in a series of articles in 2000 looking at how the media covered Mbeki and the July Durban International AIDS conference (which we cover in detail in the next chapter). Their September article by Pusch Commey, already mentioned, referred to the

> ...unrelenting media assault on the person of President Thabo Mbeki. He was variously described as irresponsible, grossly negligent and genocidal. Most thought he had lost his marbles.... The next morning's headlines [after Mbeki's opening speech] were unanimous: 'Mbeki fails to break the silence.' Then there was the usual media spin to put his speech out of context by reporting that Mbeki says the cause of Aids is poverty, while the import of his speech for those who cared to apply their minds was simply that conditions of poverty in developing countries, for which the West is a major contributor, has spawned several killer diseases, including Aids, tuberculosis, and malaria.[33]

The next month's issue had two articles analyzing in detail the media's treatment of Mbeki. Baffour Ankomah began his with the question the mainstream media were asking: "Does Mbeki suffer from 'psychological trauma?' The sharks are circling.... The prey is Thabo Mbeki, president of South Africa, the African Renaissance Man, the man who wants to see what lies at the bottom of the 'African AIDS epidemic.'" Baffour then quotes several white British and South African journalists who questioned Mbeki's sanity, answering each accusation. Then he returns to a question Mbeki had entertained:

> Now the question: If the British are promiscuous, and the majority do not use condoms, and ARE NOT catching AIDS; and if Africans are promiscuous, and the majority do not use condoms and ARE catching AIDS (as the AIDS establishment tells us), doesn't Africa deserve the right to

51

examine why the dichotomy, in order to find a cure unique to the African condition? This is what Mbeki is doing. But they say, 'No, you mustn't do that, we have the answer, the drugs and the loans here for you, take them.' Well, thank God, Africa now has, at least, one leader who is not prepared to swallow this arrogance from the North.[34]

Pusch Commey's contribution in the same issue focused on one white South African journalist, David Beresford, and his very critical piece in the British *Observer*. Commey showed in detail how articles like his "are especially notorious in the manipulation of perception at the expense of the black population." His conclusion:

> Apparently, Mr. Beresford wants President Mbeki to dispense drugs like sweets and make himself the darling of drug companies and their governments in the West. He will not. So he must be given a bad name and hanged. The 'good' black president in White South Africa/the West is the one who serves their interest at the expense of his people. Mbeki will not.[35]

Then in December, Neville Hodgkinson saw in the media treatment of Mbeki ("a new international sport... Mbeki-bashing") a reflection of the way he had been treated by the media eight years previously when he had questioned AIDS orthodoxy. The attacks on him, he said, "were emotional in tone and content," as they were against Mbeki—so that "to most newspaper readers, especially in the United States and Europe, [Mbeki] must seem monstrous.... Thanks to *New African's* coverage of the scientific controversy over AIDS, many of its readers will be aware that Mbeki has good reason for questioning the HIV story. But *New African* is a rarity... "[36]

Poverty

We have already been introduced to how the *New African* views the matter of poverty. Pusch Commey, above, noted how the media misreported Mbeki's comments on the role of poverty in causing

AIDS: "...the import of his speech *for those who cared to apply their minds* was simply that conditions of poverty in developing countries... has spawned several killer diseases, including Aids..." [emphasis mine]. Perhaps because they felt this was so obvious, the magazine did not give as much attention to this point as to some of the other points mentioned above. However, their position is clear.

In 1994, Geshekter wrote: "It is the political economy of underdevelopment, not sexual intercourse, that is killing Africans."[37] Then more than two years after Mbeki's controversial speech in Durban linking AIDS with poverty, the magazine revisited that speech by quoting from an ANC document explaining what Mbeki meant:

> Medical science everywhere in the world recognizes the central importance of diseases of poverty. Even the most highly developed countries in the world are themselves involved in a struggle against diseases of poverty. For some strange reason, Africa, among the poorest continents of the world, is not supposed to talk about these diseases of poverty and to focus on their eradication. We are urged from all sides to break the silence about HIV/Aids and maintain perfect silence about the diseases of poverty.[38]

But *New African's* most clear exposition of the link between AIDS and poverty was in an article by that name[39], written by Sam Mhlongo. Mhlongo is a South African doctor, a member of the Mbeki AIDS Panel, and generally associated with the "dissident" position. However, the assertions in his article cannot be ignored, even by orthodox scientists. He wrote:

> That tuberculosis (TB) is a disease largely associated with destitution and poverty is beyond dispute. Its prevalence diminishes as social and economic conditions improve. Sub-standard housing, shacks, and overcrowding favor the risk of massive infection or reinfection. Eighty per cent of South Africa can still be described in this way today since the inequalities of the imperialist and apartheid eras still

define the country. When one looks at the history of South Africa, it is difficult, if not impossible, not to conclude that the current debate on HIV/Aids is dominated by medicalization of diseases of poverty. Doctors and most other health professionals find it difficult, if not impossible, to deal with health-related issues without medicalizing them.

He continues:

The correlation between immunodeficiency and poverty, malnutrition, poor sanitation, urban squalor and rural and urban unemployment cannot be denied. We have now had almost 20 years of HIV/Aids, and because of the almost exclusive biomedical approach, other questions are not being asked as frequently as they should.... It is difficult in light of the evidence and the history of South Africa, to accept that a single retrovirus largely explains the disease (Aids) which doctors encounter in their practices or hospitals.

Conclusion

When I suggest to colleagues that many Africans view AIDS differently from Westerners, the response I often get is: "Well, what do they think we should do about it?" I'm caught off guard by the question. I am talking about the underlying way different people view the epidemic, and my colleagues want to talk about solutions. Clearly, the *New African* won't help them.

However, the *New African* is an excellent place to begin. It is not an academic journal nor a political party nor an activist NGO; it claims no "solutions" for the AIDS epidemic. It is simply an Afro-centric magazine that asks questions that are on the minds of many Africans. Some of those Africans, as we shall see, provide very profound analyses for some of these questions.

References

[1] **Tucker, Neely (1999):** "AIDS workers say denial, paralyzing fatalism are biggest obstacles," *Knight Ridder/Tribune News Service,* August 12.

[2] **Philpott, Paul (2000):** "Major African Magazine Reappraises HIV-AIDS Model," in *www.rethinkingaids.com/Archive/2000/RA0002NewAfrican.html.*

[3] **Philpott,** *Ibid.* **2000.**

[4] **Ankomah, Baffour and Boateng, Osei (1999),** "Knives Out For Baffour," *New African,* October.

[5] **Geshekter, Charles (1994),** "Myths of AIDS and Sex," *New African,* October.

[6] **Ankomah, Baffour (1998a),** "Monkey Business Over AIDS," *New African,* April.

[7] **Ankomah, Baffour (1999),** "AIDS Originated in the U.S. Special Virus Program," *New African,* April.

[8] **Ankomah,** *Ibid.* **1999.**

[9] *http://healtoronto.com/youngbib.html*

[10] **Boateng, Osei (2000),** "The Poison Designed to Produce an African Disease," *New African,* November.

[11] **Geshekter,** *op. cit.,* **1994.**

[12] **Christie, Huw (2000),** "The Great AIDS Debate," *New African,* May.

[13] **Chimutengwende-Gordon, Mukai (2002),** "AIDS There is Hope But," *New African,* November.

[14] **ANC Document (2002),** "Telling It As It Is," *New African,* December.

[15] **Ankomah, Baffour (2001a),** "Victory for AIDS Dissidents," *New African*, May.

[16] "Mbeki: What is the AIDS Test testing?," *New African*, June, 2001.

[17] **Ankomah, Baffour (1998b),** "Are 26 Million Africans Dying of AIDS?," *New African*, December.

[18] **Fiala, Christian (1998),** "Dirty Tricks Over AIDS Figures," *New African*, April.

[19] **Ankomah,** *op. cit.,* **1998b.**

[20] **Boateng, Osei, and Offei-Ansah, Jon (2002),** "'No Blood-Based Study on AIDS Conducted,'" *New African*, April.

[21] **ANC Document,** *op. cit.* **2002.**

[22] **Fiala,** *op. cit.* **1998.**

[23] **Ankomah,** *op. cit.,* **1998b.**

[24] **Ankomah, Baffour (2001b),** "AIDS: Rhetoric and Reality," *New African*, March.

[25] **Ankomah,** *op. cit.,* **1998b.**

[26] **Ankomah,** *op. cit.,* **2001b.**

[27] **Banda, Muzondwa (1999a),** "AIDS: Let Them Eat Their Figures," *New African*, September.

[28] **Banda, Muzondwa (1999b),** "Mbeki's AIDS Bombshell," *New African*, December.

[29] **Christie,** *op. cit.,* **2000.**

[30] **Commey, Pusch (2000a),** "AIDS: Judgment Day on the 13th," *New African*, September.

[31] **Boateng, Osei (2001)**, "The Profits That Kill," *New African*, April.

[32] **Ankomah and Boateng**, *op. cit.*, **1999**.

[33] **Commey**, *op. cit.*, **2000**.

[34] **Ankomah, Baffour (2000)**, "Baffour's Beefs," *New African*, October.

[35] **Commey, Pusch (2000b)**, "Opinion," *New African*, October.

[36] **Hodgkinson, Neville (2000)**, "Viewpoint: 'Eight years ago, I went through the same experience as Mbeki,'" *New African*, December.

[37] **Geshekter**, *op. cit.*, **1994**.

[38] **ANC Document**, *op. cit.*, **2002**.

[39] **Mhlongo, Sam (2001),** "Aids and Poverty: Doctors in Africa appear to have forgotten that many of the sick they encounter have always satisfied the Bangui definition of Aids," *New African*, July-August.

3

Thabo Mbeki:
The Flashpoint of the African AIDS Discourse

Probably no single person has influenced the discourse of AIDS in Africa as much as Thabo Mbeki, the president of South Africa. Certainly no one has been as controversial. Even as I write, news articles still refer to Mbeki as the one who was slow to respond to his country's AIDS crisis, and who formerly even questioned the link between HIV and AIDS. These articles generally point out that Mbeki's government has made a "turn-around" — the implication being that Mbeki was wrong, and has now either changed his mind or bowed to the pressure of those who are "right". There are no suggestions that he may have been misunderstood, no admission that he was on the right track, no questioning of the conventional wisdom of the West which says, as US President George W. Bush said, "We know how to prevent AIDS, and we know how to treat it."[1] For the Western media, Mbeki's views on AIDS are history — and wrong.

However, one of the more striking aspects of the Mbeki AIDS Story is the difference between the way he was viewed in Africa and the way he was interpreted by the Western media. As noted above, the Western media generally crucified him. The South African media were mixed. But in the rest of Africa, most of what I read and heard about Mbeki and his views on AIDS was positive. For those of us concerned about AIDS in Africa, it is crucial to consider this difference, to try and understand how Mbeki's speeches and actions can be seen so differently by different people.

October 1998 to April 2000

The story of Thabo Mbeki's involvement with his country's AIDS epidemic begins during the administration of Nelson Mandela, when Mbeki was Deputy President. Despite the rapidly growing number of South African AIDS cases in the late 90s, the Mandela administration did not take a public stance on the problem, being preoccupied with holding the country together in those first five years after the fall of Apartheid. It did not ignore AIDS, however; there was an ill-fated attempt to educate about the disease in an expensive but unsuccessful musical, *Sarafina II*, and later Mandela's party, the African National Congress, (ANC) threw its weight behind an experimental but ultimately bogus drug for AIDS treatment called Virodene. Future critics of Mbeki would point to these early failed attempts, which Mbeki was involved in, to bolster their case that Mbeki was inept, or even dangerous, when he dealt with AIDS.

Mbeki's first speech on the disease, however, did not support this theory. On Friday, October 9, 1998, Mandela was scheduled to give a major policy speech on AIDS, and had ordered the country's flags flown at half mast to remember those who had already died of the disease. However, Mandela was indisposed, so he asked his Deputy President Mbeki to speak instead. The speech Mbeki gave was brief, succinct, and (in light of the subsequent controversy) remarkably non-controversial. Central to it was the "ABC approach"[2] of Uganda: Abstain, Be faithful, use Condoms:

> But I appeal to the young people, who represent our country's future, to abstain from sex for as long as possible. If you decide to engage in sex, use a condom. In the same way, I appeal to both men and women to be faithful to each other, but otherwise to use condoms.

This advice was preceded by the statement that "HIV spreads mainly through sex" — note he refers not just to the disease AIDS, but to the virus HIV.[3] The speech was entirely conventional.

Six months later Mbeki was elected President of South Africa — and won by a greater margin than Mandela had. But the controversy about the South African AIDS policy had already begun. Before Mbeki's election, the Ministry of Health of Mandela's administration had decided to stop a pilot project, which was giving the drug AZT to pregnant women who were HIV positive in a bid to stop the transmission of the virus to the infant. The government said the drug was too expensive. On November 1, 1998, the Global News Wire released two articles criticizing the decision.[4]

A year later, the problem hadn't been solved. Mbeki, now president, was concerned as well about the toxicity of AZT. In mid-November, 1999, the new Minister of Health, Dr. M. E. Tshabalala-Msimang, presented a lengthy statement to the National Assembly, almost half of it dealing systematically with her concerns about using AZT for preventing mother-to-child transmission (MTCT) of HIV. She reviewed several studies about the effectiveness AZT, and a newer drug nevirapine, given to HIV positive pregnant women to prevent transmission of the virus to the infant. She reminded the audience that not all infants born to HIV positive mothers become infected with the virus—only 25%. She also explained that the drugs were effective only one third to one half of the time, especially when the women continued breast-feeding—and that long-term toxicities were unknown. Some rats given high doses of AZT eventually developed vaginal cancer—the same long-term side effect eventually found in some girls whose mothers were given stilbesterol when they were in utero. She concluded that there was not yet enough information available to assure the "affordability and appropriateness" of continuing the AZT program for preventing mother-to-child transmission.[5]

To put this decision in perspective, it is important to consider the standard of care in the rest of Africa. Most countries in Africa have a national health system which owns and runs hospitals, employs their staff, and provides the running costs. There are other systems, mostly private and mission, but they are usually more costly, and most Africans do not have health insurance. Small government hospitals have limited formularies, and rarely carry anti-cancer drugs, expensive antibiotics, or the latest cardiac drugs. Many of these drugs would be available at larger private hospitals or in the capital cities. In 1998-9, at the time South Africa decided to suspend an AZT pilot program, few other African countries were using anti-retrovirals, the class of anti-AIDS drugs to which AZT belongs. They were not "forbidden" or outlawed by the governments; they were simply too expensive for government hospitals to buy.

It is also important to consider the particular situation of controversy then in South Africa. The use of anti-AIDS drugs to treat AIDS, which then cost about US$10,000 a year for the three drugs necessary, was not really being debated anywhere in Africa. It was far too costly. (This debate would eventually occur, as we shall see at the end of this chapter.) What was being debated was the use of a single drug given to pregnant women and then to their newborn infants to reduce the transmission of HIV to the infant. As Dr. Tshabalala-Msimang pointed out, less than one third of the babies born to HIV positive mothers will get the virus, and the drugs are effective less than half the time. This means that of 100 HIV positive pregnant women given AZT, the infants of fewer than 17 would benefit. What has been repeatedly called "genocide"[6] was really this: deciding not to pay for—but not outlawing—a drug with unknown long-term side effects that could have prevented a small percentage of infant HIV infections, and none of the adult infections.

Is 17% a small percent? In the West, 17 "preventable" deaths out of 100 is not small; 83 people out of 100 taking a drug that does not help them is not unreasonable. But we conclude this based on current Western medical standards and ethics. Are these standards and ethics universal? Prof. Jesse Mugambi, who we quoted in the introduction ("Interpreting African life using foreign norms as the criteria... will distort the real nature of African life"), also says this: "...patronizing foreigners... feel that what their civilized culture has selected as the best way of life is necessarily also the best way of life for Africans."[7] Mbeki's Minister of Health was questioning that assumption.

By early 2000, Mbeki became very interested in the AIDS problem, and read extensively about it. He saw a discrepancy between how AIDS was being described by conventional scientists, and what he was seeing in his own country. In raising questions about this difference, he became aware of the views of the so-called dissident scientists who doubted that HIV caused AIDS, but felt other factors such as poverty were more important. He invited several of these dissidents, along with twice as many conventional scientists, to be on a panel to discuss the nature of the African epidemic.

The world media clearly did not approve of his approach. *The New York Times* published an article on March 19 titled "South Africa in a Furor Over Advice About AIDS"[8], and on April 1 the British medical journal *Lancet* gave voice to some opponents of Mbeki. One said "Mbeki has given lifeblood to a dead cause.... It's tantamount to Holocaust denial..."; another that it was a "national scandal"; and still others that he is "undermining the efforts of AIDS-awareness campaigns."[9] The conclusion of the *British Medical Journal*, backed up by *no* quotes from Mbeki himself, was that "Mbeki believes that AIDS is not caused by HIV."[10]

It was at this point in the debate, April 3, 2000, that Mbeki sent a letter to many world leaders, explaining his position. He said, in part,

Accordingly, as Africans, we have to deal with this uniquely African catastrophe that:

- contrary to the West, HIV-AIDS in Africa is heterosexually transmitted;

- contrary to the West, where relatively few people have died from AIDS, itself a matter of serious concern, millions are said to have died in Africa; and,

- contrary to the West, where AIDS deaths are declining, even greater numbers of Africans are destined to die.

It is obvious that whatever lessons we have to and may draw from the West about the grave issue of HIV-AIDS, a simple superimposition of Western experience on African reality would be absurd and illogical. Such proceeding would constitute a criminal betrayal of our responsibility to our own people.... I am convinced that our urgent task is to respond to the specific threat that faces us as Africans. We will not eschew this obligation in favors of the comfort of the recitation of a catechism that may very well be a correct response to the specific manifestation of AIDS in the West. We will not, ourselves, condemn our own people to death by giving up the search for specific and targeted responses to the specifically African incidence of HIV-AIDS.[11]

The Western press was not impressed. On Wednesday, April 19, *The Washington Post* published a copy of the letter, and in another article that day reported that several officials in the Clinton administration "expressed dismay at Mbeki's decision to intensify what they see as a diversionary dispute..."[12] The next day in the same newspaper was an editorial calling Mbeki's position "a dangerous denial" — while ironically accurately describing some reasons why anti-viral drugs would be difficult to sustain in nations like South Africa ("... life-extending drugs are too costly to make them usable. Even if drug prices were to fall, the infrastructure for distribution does not exist.").[13]

It is at this point that we begin to see the articulation of African views. On April 26, 2000, *The Nation* of Kenya published a lengthy article supporting Mbeki's letter. However, unlike the Western reports, the *Nation* article did not focus on Mbeki's association with the dissidents. This was the core of the *Nation* argument:

> ... The question on the minds of many people is what could possibly be wrong with seeking alternative approaches to the HIV/Aids problem. Africans, ravaged as they are by this pandemic, have for long remained completely helpless in the face of Western effusiveness and intellectual arrogance on HIV/Aids. After blaming the continent, without any substantive evidence, for having been the origin of the HIV virus, Western pundits have gone ahead to frustrate any attempts by African thinkers to contribute to anti-HIV efforts. A century of Western medicine has, to a large extent, incapacitated large segments of the human race and made millions of people dependent on daily doses of what can easily pass for poison. Indeed, the line between pharmaceutical drugs and poison is very thin. Modern medicine's failure to find a cure for diseases such

as cancer, malaria and now, HIV/Aids, is a severe indictment of Western medicine's efficacy as the sole provider of cures for human ailments. As a result of imbibing Western medical edicts, knowledge of traditional African medicine has been thrown to the dogs. Herbalists are considered an anachronism and their trade quackery...[14]

The author then touched on the role of pharmaceutical companies and patents, matters which would occupy the headlines in South Africa a year later.

INTERLUDE I—Germs and Drugs

At first, this African view sounds like an overstated, paranoid view of the risks of pharmaceuticals, a view we can easily dismiss. However, these opinions look more sensible when we consider them in the context of a brief history of pharmacology.

We treat most diseases with drugs—to cure, to ameliorate, or even to prevent. Historically, traditional healers have gone to the forest or garden to find herbs and leaves and roots and bark that gave relief to the symptoms of disease, sometimes even eliminating it. Eventually that task was taken over by pharmacists, and more recently by pharmaceutical companies which manufacture the drugs. But the underlying concept of using plant substances to treat disease is ancient.

Obviously we need a method to decide *which* drugs to use for which diseases—and we have one. Louise Lander, in discussing modern Western medicine, says

The theoretical core of modern medical ideology is the germ theory of disease: the notion that particular microscopic agents are the sole cause of particular illnesses.... The germ theory of disease has found a generalized form in the doctrine of specific etiology, or causation: the notion that a given disease can be explained by a distinct, well-defined biochemical or physiologic abnormality. The whole theoretical and finally ideological superstructure is commonly known as the biomedical model.... The biomedical model has provided the ideological underpinnings of, and has in turn been nourished by, the activities of the biomedical research establishment and the drug industry in their development of modern medicine's enormous armamentarium of medications: 'Whatever the nature of the disease, the most important task—so at least is the well-nigh universal belief—is to discover some magic bullet capable of reaching and destroying the responsible demon within the body of the patient.'[15]

Our method, in other words, is to find the bug, then find a drug that will kill that bug. The method seems simple and straight-forward. However, disease is not always that simple or straight-forward. The biomedical model is only one way to understand disease, and it is limited. It contains:

...the general assumption that disease reflects disordered biological mechanisms that can ultimately be described in terms of chemistry and physics and that are independent of social behavior or intrapsychic processes. The model is reductionistic, explaining complex phenomena by invoking a single ultimate principle; dualistic, reflecting a separation of mind and body; and mechanistic, reflecting a view of the human body as a machine.

Treatment, therefore, focuses "on defeating the microbe rather than on altering the environment so as to strengthen the resistance of the host."

Drugs do work, at least partially. But their success should not prohibit a critique of this approach, which gained ascendancy a century ago. Louise Lander again: "For the medical practitioners the germ theory was much more serviceable than the environmental approach to the treatment of illness, for it justified their one-to-one relationships with members of the upper classes, whose living and working environments were in any event less unhealthy than those of the poor." An approach that focused more on the intra-psychic and external environments would threaten "the vested interests that are protected by the biomedical model.... The pharmaceutical industry would not only lose a customer in the immediate sense but would possibly also lose a participant in the lifelong symbiotic relationship with that industry that most people enter into, much to its profit."

We can begin to see here some common ground with what we have heard from the Kenyan *Nation* author above—and certainly from Mbeki. While never denying the germ that was involved with AIDS, Mbeki emphasized that the environment—poverty—was a far larger reason for ill health in Africa. His approach earned him few friends at the Durban meeting of scientists, as we shall soon see, a meeting financed in part by the pharmaceutical industry.

> To the medical care system and to the larger political economy, a major usefulness of the technological, market commodity, curative definition of medical care is that it obscures the social origin of so many ills—their roots in the social order—and diverts attention from the social interventions that would constitute real change.[16]

This broad understanding of medicine, though not in vogue today among researchers, is certainly not unique to the authors just quoted. Rudolf Virchow in the mid-19th Century concluded that "the physician had to concern himself with the total environment of human beings and therefore could not avoid taking part in political action."[17] In the 1970s and 80s, several authors critically explored what they called the "role of medicine", many following the ideas of Rene Dubos in his 1959 *Mirage of Health,* and concluded that the influence of medicine on health may be less important than we have assumed.[18] A characteristic sentiment is this: "... medical expertise may often be misapplied and even wrong in respect of the explanations it offers and the treatments it recommends."[19] These critiques provide an excellent foundation for the "maverick" position that Mbeki has taken. Why, then—some might ask—did he consult the dissidents of the 90s instead of this more "respectable" body of knowledge?

There are a few obvious reasons: These authors did not refer to AIDS—they were all writing before it was an epidemic. None focused their analysis on Africa. They are more obscure, and none of them have internet sites. And possibly Mbeki would not see the connections I have just outlined. The distance between their world and Mbeki's was simply too great.

However, there is an uncomfortable assumption hidden in this question of who Mbeki consulted. Most news reports referred to him "associating with" or "flirting with" dissidents, "seeking their advice", "aligning himself" with them, "adopting" their views— though the media did not use these terms of association for Mbeki's relationship with the two-thirds of the Panel that were conventional "orthodox" scientists. But a few media reports said openly what the others only implied: that Mbeki was "tempted by," "inspired by," and even "seduced by" the dissidents. Some pointed to the irony of him seeking American advice for his African solutions. All of this reporting assumes that Mbeki had few ideas of his own, and that eccentric thinkers filled his mind with nonsense. The same media admit confusion as to why an otherwise intelligent educated African leader would allow himself to be duped.

There is another way to understand Mbeki. Likely, instead of having no philosophy of disease and treatment, he had an African philosophy deeply rooted in his consciousness. And likely, when he saw the responses of the scientific community to the AIDS epidemic, he felt a dissonance with his African understanding. The dissidents also felt a dissonance, and for a while he found himself on the same path as them. But Mbeki himself is not a "dissident" in the Western sense—that is, a "denialist"; he is, as he claimed in his now famous May 8, 1996 speech, an African.

"What this means," he said elsewhere, "is that we must recall everything that is good and inspiring in our past.... As every revolution requires revolutionaries, so must the African renaissance have its militants and activists who will define the morrow that belongs to them in a way which will help to restore us to our dignity.... Our first task, therefore, is to transform our society consistent with this vision..."[20] Very likely, Mbeki's broad understanding of AIDS was part of this vision, and his militancy was his stubborn defense of it.

The Panel

In case anyone still had doubts about what Mbeki believed about the HIV virus, he made his views clear on May 22, 2000 during a US interview on The NewsHour With Jim Lehrer.[21] The interviewer Gwen Ifill asked, "... You've said that you were mischaracterized in some of the comments you said about the relationship between HIV and AIDS... Exactly where do you stand with that now do you think?"

Mbeki responded, "Well, yes, I don't know where these reports came from, that we're taking a position saying there's no connection from HIV—between HIV and AIDS. I never said it..." She then asked about his opposition to AZT, and he told her his reasons: "Affordability, medical infrastructure in order to dispense these medicines, [and] potential toxicity." In the same interview he explained why he invited the dissident scientists, explained again the difference between the African and American epidemics, and explained his desire to confront AIDS together with all the other health problems facing South Africa.

He had said essentially the same thing during his introductory remarks to the first meeting of the presidential Advisory Panel on Aids in Pretoria, May 6, 2000. Reviewing his own understanding until that point, he said: "What we knew was that there is a virus, HIV. The virus causes AIDS." He then asked the Panel members to consider why that virus seemed to be acting so differently in Africa compared to the West.[22]

What Mbeki was asking of this particular group was very difficult. Based on some questions he had about the appropriateness of the mainstream scientific approach to AIDS, he invited prominent scientists who had reached quite different conclusions to talk with each other. He was looking for scientific answers that could deal with what he clearly felt was a "catastrophe" in his country. But more than that: he realized that the pattern of AIDS in South Africa had rapidly changed from a Western pattern—primarily in homosexual men and intravenous drug users—to a heterosexually transmitted pattern, a change that had not occurred in the West. He wanted to know how this could be explained scientifically.

But why invite this particular group of scientists? Why include the very small but vocal group of dissidents? The answer is fairly obvious. One of the dissidents on the Panel, Dr. Peter Duesberg, had previously suggested that instead of being caused by a virus, AIDS was caused perhaps by toxins, or poor nutrition. Commenting later on the panel itself, Duesberg reviewed some of his own recommendations: "... invest money, if there is such money, into improving the standard of living, like nutrition and sanitation and health standards, conventional health care."[23] Mbeki knew that a better standard of living and nutrition and sanitation and conventional health care were all important in the fight against AIDS, and now he was hearing a PhD scientist who was recommending these very things. He wanted to hear more. His goal was to combine the best of the dissident suggestions— dissidents made up about one third of the panel—with the conventional wisdom of the other two thirds.

There are reports of what actually happened in the Panel from at least seven people who were there—five panel members[24][25][26][27] and two journalists[28][29]—half of them mainstream and half dissident. Their reports are quite helpful in letting us see how a panel like this failed to reach any consensus. People from both "sides" agreed that there were clearly sides, and that no real dialogue took place. But the failure of the Panel to honestly address the question Mbeki was asking does not invalidate the question.

Maybe Mbeki invited the wrong people; maybe biomedical scientists should not be expected to advise on policy. Results of scientific research may indeed be key drivers of public policy, as the final Panel Report suggested, but does that policy flow directly from the results? As we saw above, the biomedical model of understanding disease, though quite "accurate", does not always tell us what to do about that disease. Or maybe the Panel and the news media focused on the wrong question: settling the viral question may not be necessary in order to fight against the disease.

But the scientific community thought that *was* the key question. Responding to the "threat" posed by a dozen or so dissident scientists, over 5,000 conventional scientists signed a "Durban Declaration" that was published in the journal *Nature* as the Panel was meeting for the second time, just a week before the beginning of the XIII International Aids Conference in Durban. The Declaration was intended to lay to rest the question of etiology by declaring that the HIV virus, the virus alone, caused AIDS.[30]

One final note about this viral debate: although about one-third of those on the Panel were black Africans, virtually all of those who published their perceptions of the Panel were white and not from South Africa. A few months after the panel met M. S. Prabhakara, writing in *The Hindu* of India, suggested that the entire AIDS debate in South Africa remained Eurocentric. "Indeed," he wrote, "in the whole HIV/AIDS controversy, one looks in vain for any reference to the literature outside what continues to be South Africa's spiritual homeland—England and the United States and the broad Anglo-American alliance." He concluded with a reference to "the more fundamental Eurocentrism mindset that continues to set the agenda in South Africa—notwithstanding all the hype about an African renaissance."[31] Although as we have seen and will see further, Africans have been contributing to the HIV/AIDS controversy all along, the contributors to the South African debate up to this point were mostly Western. Except, of course, Mbeki.

The Durban Aids Conference

On July 9, 2000, the world media gave Mbeki a test. According to most he failed—and that failure, in their eyes, has yet to be overturned. He was giving the opening speech at the XIII International AIDS Conference, held for the first time on the African continent. Everyone knew about the Panel; everyone wanted Mbeki to declare, as the Durban Declaration did, that HIV was the sole, undisputed cause of AIDS. But Mbeki did not feel that that was what this audience needed to hear. Never in his speech did he deny the existence and importance of the virus; throughout, in fact, he referred to "HIV and AIDS" or "HIV-AIDS". What Mbeki emphasized instead was the importance of poverty as a substrate for the AIDS spread in Africa. Then, comparing what the World Health Organization had said about the importance of poverty with what he was hearing about the importance of the HIV virus, he said,

> As I listened and heard the whole story told about our own country, it seemed to me that we could not blame everything on a single virus. It seemed to me also that every living African, whether in good or ill- health, is prey to many enemies of health that would interact one upon the other in many ways, within one human body. And thus I came to conclude that we have a desperate and pressing need to wage a war on all fronts to guarantee and realize the human right of all our people to good health. And so, being insufficiently educated, and therefore ill-prepared to answer this question, I started to ask the question, expecting an answer from others, what is to be done, particularly about HIV-AIDS! One of the questions I have asked is, 'are safe sex, condoms and anti-retroviral drugs a sufficient response to the health catastrophe we face?'[32]

Among the audience of 12,000 people, some apparently did not like what they were hearing. While Mbeki spoke about poverty to this "large crowd of mostly white, mostly foreign researchers, doctors, and AIDS activists,"[33] some called out "what about HIV?"[34], and others that his views had "nothing to do with our lives."[35] Hundreds, according to the *Washington Post*, walked out on his speech "when he failed to renounce his skepticism about what causes the disease and how it is treated."[36]

In other words, some in the audience—including the media—had a clear idea of what they expected Mbeki to say, but it was his speech, not theirs. He did not satisfy their expectations. While never denying the essence of the orthodox view, he was offering his audience a chance to view the AIDS epidemic more broadly; they were offering him a chance to articulate their "correct" narrow view. The 12,000, with their media in tow, saw to it that the narrow view would be proclaimed the loudest.

However, Mbeki was not utterly alone. Simon Barber of the Johannesburg *Business Day* was disgusted by what he called the "lazy journalist virus" that dominated the media coverage of Mbeki's speech.[37] "Monday morning's US media accounts of President Thabo Mbeki's opening address to the 13th international AIDS conference in Durban," he wrote, "were proof of the lazily thought-free pack mentality of much of the journalistic profession, especially when it comes to sensitive and complicated issues." After reviewing some of the negative coverage, he quoted from several "orthodox" sources—including the Durban Declaration meant to oppose Mbeki—that "co-factors" were important in the spread of AIDS. Then he quoted from Mbeki's speech, showing how he was saying the same thing. "The critics," he continued, "would like him to focus exclusively on HIV/AIDS, stemming its transmission and treating the infected. He said, yes, we must discourage dangerous behavior, care for its victims and search for vaccine, but as part of a holistic effort to improve public health and living standards, and reduce the poverty which happens to be a breeding ground for AIDS cofactors."

"Listen to Mbeki, Durban delegates," he concluded. "The AIDS crisis in Africa must be treated holistically. The cofactors are as important a target as the HIV bug. Remember the dictum of Louis Pasteur: 'the terrain is as important as the germ.' Will you self-interestedly focus on the germ or will you heed Mbeki's call to help cleanse the terrain?"

After the Durban AIDS conference, media coverage of Mbeki increased in Europe and America, and most of it did not take this advice. Just for an example: The *Guardian Weekly* began their coverage with a July 6 article entitled "Scientists denounce Mbeki's 'Aids error'", followed the week after by a front page article, "HIV judge berates Mbeki for Aids confusion". The week after again it was, "Mandela unites Africa in battle against HIV"—interpreting Mandela's support of new drug treatments as a "coded message to... Mbeki" not to delay their introduction into South Africa. On August 24, there was an article entitled "Mbeki faces court battle on Aids drug" which included a reference to Mbeki "letting babies die". By September 28 the *Guardian* quoted several South African leaders opposed to Mbeki's position in "Friends turn on Mandela's faltering heir".

There was, however, another more sympathetic point of view being articulated after the Durban conference. These voices, mostly from Africans in Africa, were remarkably consistent in their affirmation of what Mbeki was saying. They were not loud, and certainly not organized or coordinated; consequently the consistency of their message went virtually unnoticed by the Western press. It is therefore ironic that a few of these were recorded by that media. For example, the first *Washington Post* article to report on the Durban conference—the one that reported that hundreds had walked out on Mbeki's speech—quoted Abraham Alabi, "a 40-year-old Nigerian microbiologist working in Gambia": "Mbeki's speech, I think, is very truthful, linking poverty to so many of these diseases."[38] It was a single, quiet voice, drowned out by the chorus of protest the *Post* was reporting on.

Two weeks later the *Science Magazine* quoted David Serwadda of Makerere University in Uganda regarding the clamor to import anti-aids drugs: he was concerned that drug-resistant viruses would proliferate if patients did not adhere to the complicated treatment regimens. He had good reason to be concerned: "HIV treatment 'can't be any easier than tuberculosis, and we have 35% failure with TB.'"[39] It was another quiet, extremely important—and ignored—voice. TB treatment is usually for 6 months with three drugs that are less toxic than anti-AIDS drugs, and they are often supplied free in Africa. Anti-aids drugs are more toxic, need to be monitored more closely, are far more expensive, and need to be taken for the rest of one's life. If the relatively simple TB treatment has 35% failure, has anyone asked why? Have they considered what the failure rate might be for anti-AIDS drugs, not to mention the resistant strains that would undoubtedly develop?

Not surprisingly, the African news media were a much better place to find the African voices. Before the Durban conference began, Timothy Kalyegira reported from Uganda that "South Africa calls for African approach to AIDS."[40] On July 15, *The Dispatch* from Accra, Ghana titled their article "South Africa: Controversy at AIDS Forum", but reported on Mbeki's position this way: he "said poverty, and not AIDS, was the most dangerous threat to the people of Africa," and "that HIV is not wholly responsible for AIDS."[41] A few days later, the *New Vision* of Uganda published a brief article in which Dr Tshabalala-Msimang, the South Africa Minister of Health, clarified Mbeki's position on AIDS: he "did not say that HIV does not cause AIDS as recently reported," but she emphasized "that the AIDS problem could not be solved by looking at HIV alone" — again referring to the need to confront poverty.[42]

The next month Allehone Mulugeta published a lengthy commentary on the AIDS debate in the *Addis Tribune* of Addis Ababa, Ethiopia. He said "Mr. Mbeki is urging Africans to transcend their limitations and rethink the basics of the disease... [W]hat he is doing is a logical outworking of a leadership culture that is built on strong political will to make a difference to the constituency" — likely a reference to his earlier anti-apartheid work. Yet "in asking the basics he played the unorthodox and was attacked both by the media and the medical gurus..."[43]

At the end of August there was an "alternative" international AIDS conference in Uganda, which we will look at in detail in the next chapter. Although "dissident" scientists organized it and gave their opinions, most of the African presenters did not enter the debate about etiology at all, but rather used Mbeki's views as a starting point to explore their distinctly African understandings of the epidemic. Their analyses were profound — and completely missed by the media.

In September, the *New African* Magazine did their major story on Mbeki and the Durban conference, an article we referred to in the last chapter. The article began by discussing the "unrelenting media assault" on Mbeki that preceded the conference, then reviewed the conference itself. Concerning Mbeki's opening speech, "the next morning's headlines were unanimous: 'Mbeki fails to break the silence.' Then there was the usual media spin to put his speech out of context by reporting that Mbeki says the cause of AIDS is poverty, while the import of his speech for those who cared to apply their minds was simply that conditions of poverty in developing countries, for which the West is a major contributor, has spawned several killer diseases, including AIDS, tuberculosis and malaria. And that to make any impact, the world must attack the conditions that create poverty."

Later in the month, Sam Mwale in *The East African* revisited a question that many Africans feel is very important: Did AIDS really originate in Africa? And if so, how? "During the Durban conference," he wrote, "a lot of energy was spent denouncing efforts to find and understand the origins of Aids. Conventional wisdom seems to be that all efforts should focus on developing and implementing effective preventive and, when technology will allow, curative measures. While the latter position is sensible given the grim consequences of the pandemic, it does not diminish the moral and legal responsibility of that same establishment to get to the bottom of the mystery of the source and origin of Aids." He felt that Mbeki's "line of inquiry may help Africa get to the bottom of how HIV came to infect humans, and Africans in particular."[44]

Not all African reports, naturally, fell in lock step behind Mbeki. *This Day* in Lagos, Nigeria, reported in October, "South African Doctors Fault Mbeki's View on HIV/AIDS" and quoted the doctors' Chairman, Zolile Mlisana: "'HIV does cause AIDS. It is not a matter of political opinion. President Mbeki is wrong if he implies doubt about HIV causing AIDS.'" But even this "negative" African view of Mbeki was not wholly negative. The article ended this way:

> The chairman however agreed with Mbeki's position on seeking non-medical measures to prevent the spread of the disease, especially in cases of medical disasters and epidemics, adding that in those areas it was important to note and emphasize that these are not arrested by the administration of medicines, but by social reengineering, prevention and public health measures. In this regard, Mlisana said Mbeki was right if he was attempting to force

doctors to consider more than just the virus and administration of medicines on the issue of HIV/AIDS.[45]

Almost the same message came from the Panafrica News Agency article, "Kenyan Doctor Defends Mbeki on AIDS". Dr. Obuogo Subiri,

> who was present at the [Durban] conference, said the Western media misinterpreted Mbeki's speech, which blamed poverty rather than HIV, the virus believed to cause AIDS, as the main enemy and cause of the spread of HIV/AIDS, especially in Africa. '[President] Mbeki did not intend to throw into confusion the link between HIV and AIDS, and this confusion was exacerbated by the Western media.... The message that came out of his [President Mbeki's] speech was not that people should stop using condoms as has been alleged, and I strongly believe Mbeki wanted to affirm that we must fight poverty first in order to tackle AIDS,' he added.[46]

Mbeki's Interviews

In general, then, following the Panel and the Durban AIDS Conference, media coverage of the Mbeki AIDS story fell into two categories. The loudest voices came from the wealthier Western media, including South African media; these were mostly critical of his position (except for Simon Barber), assuming he was denying any link between HIV and AIDS, as well as denying the extent of the AIDS problem in South Africa. The quieter voices (summarized in some detail above) came mostly from the African media; these generally saw value in what Mbeki was saying, and tried to interpret him to their readers. These opposing opinions, however, did not generally lead to confusion, except possibly in South Africa itself. In the rest of Africa, people thought Mbeki was right; in the West, they thought he was wrong.

Unfortunately, the few times that Mbeki was interviewed by the mainstream press did not bring clarity. It is worth looking carefully at these interviews to see why. The European edition of *Time* Magazine published an interview with Mbeki in their September 11, 2000 issue. This was part of their conversation about AIDS:

> *TIME:* "You've been criticized for playing down the link between HIV and AIDS. Where do you now stand on this very controversial issue?"
>
> **Mbeki:** "Clearly there is such a thing as acquired immune deficiency. The question you have to ask is what produces this deficiency. A whole variety of things can cause the immune system to collapse. Now it is perfectly possible that among those things is a particular virus. But the notion that immune deficiency is only acquired from a single virus cannot be sustained. Once you say immune deficiency is acquired from that virus your response will be antiviral drugs. But if you accept that there can be a variety of reasons, including poverty and the many diseases that afflict Africans, then you can have a more comprehensive treatment response."
>
> *TIME:* "Are you prepared to acknowledge that there is a link between HIV and AIDS?"
>
> **Mbeki:** "No, I am saying that you cannot attribute immune deficiency solely and exclusively to a virus. There may very well be a virus.... But if you come to the conclusion that the only thing that destroys immune systems is HIV then your only response is to give them antiretroviral drugs.... If the scientists ... say this virus is part of the variety of things from which people acquire immune deficiency, I have no problem with that."[47]

Following this interview, the South African Government Communication and Information Service (GCIS) tried to clarify the resulting confusion:

> ... the published edited version in *Time*, on which many critics now depend, conflated his remarks in a way which could give rise to a misunderstanding over his (generic or non-specific) use of the word 'no' after being asked if he was prepared to acknowledge that there was a link between HIV and AIDS. In fact, the President went on to say that 'you cannot attribute immune deficiency *solely and exclusively* to a virus'. The context of the full transcript

77

makes it expressly clear that he was prepared to accept
that HIV might 'very well' be a causal factor...[48]

As the GCIS points out, it is clear that Mbeki *does* see a link between
HIV and AIDS. His "no" was likely a refusal to be limited to the
"doctrine of specific etiology" mentioned in the Germs and Drugs
"Interlude" above. His "no" was an affirmation that "the terrain is
as important as the germ" — the wisdom of Pasteur that Simon
Barber reminded us of.

When we realize that Mbeki was speaking from this broader
understanding of disease causation, another puzzling interview
begins to make sense – one we quoted from in the previous
chapter. On April 24, 2001, he was interviewed on South African
television.

> **Debra Patta:** "President Mbeki, HIV/AIDS has dominated the
> headlines in South Africa for the last two years and bit before
> that as well, let's bring this down to the personal level – would
> you take an HIV/AIDS test?"
>
> **Mbeki:** "Sitting where I sit as the President of South Africa, I
> think that the challenge I face is to have all outstanding questions
> with regard to this matter answered so that we are then able to
> respond as effectively as possible to the AIDS challenge. So the
> matter of whether I take an HIV test or not, I think is irrelevant to
> the matter. It might be dramatic, and make newspaper
> headlines."
>
> **Patta** (interrupts): "But would it not set an example – the
> president takes an AIDS test?"
>
> **Mbeki:** "No, but it would be setting an example within the
> context of a particular paradigm.... Now I don't believe that
> stunts — publicity stunts — help in addressing the health needs of
> our people.... The panel said one of things we have got to do is to
> determine when you do an HIV test what is the test testing. And
> those were the scientists: what is it measuring. So I go and do a
> test I'm confirming a particular paradigm. It doesn't help in
> addressing this health need. Our focus must be how do we
> improve the health of our people and that is what we are focused
> on."[49]

The paradigm that Mbeki was referring to was the "doctrine of specific etiology". This paradigm says that when we find *the* germ that causes a disease; all we need to do is find *the* drug or drugs to fight that germ. That approach is not only reductionistic, but also biased toward pharmacological responses to disease. In another context, Mbeki said,

> [I]f one agrees that HIV causes AIDS, then it follows that the condition must be treated with drugs, and those drugs are produced by the big Western drug companies; these drug companies therefore need HIV to cause AIDS, so they promote the thesis that HIV causes AIDS;... drug companies were only interested in developing medicines to combat a disease if they could make a profit out of that disease.[50]

The broader paradigm that Mbeki speaks from clearly has room for germs and drugs; in his *Time* interview he accepted that "this virus is part of the variety of things from which people acquire immune deficiency," and referred to "a more comprehensive treatment response" which could clearly include drugs. But he was not willing to focus solely on the HIV virus and antiretroviral drugs — and neither should we.

There is one more interview worth considering. On August 6, 2001, Tim Sebastian of the BBC interviewed Mbeki. Parts of the transcript sounded simply like an argument between the two. However, there were a few interchanges in the middle of this argument which some people feel is at the heart of the problem of the Mbeki controversy. For example:

> **Tim Sebastian:** "AIDS workers in Soweto have said you have damaged the campaign [against AIDS]; you've muddied the waters..."
> **Thabo Mbeki:** "I think that's a load of nonsense."
> **TS:** "Even the head of your Trade Union movement says, you know, that this can undermine the message that all South Africans must take precautions to avoid infection."
> **TM:** "Nonsense, absolute nonsense..."

And a bit later in the interview:

> **TS:** "I wonder whether you realize, whether you accept that your position has actually damaged the fight against AIDS in this country."
> **TM:** "I don't."

And still later in the interview:

> **TM:** "... in your approach to AIDS you've got to go beyond the question, merely, of a virus."
> **TS:** "But people say that you now have men sitting around saying TM says we don't need condoms, we don't need ..., we don't need to protect ourselves because there's no link between HIV and AIDS."
> **TM:** "No that's not true..."
> **TS:** "But that's the effect..."
> **TM:** "It isn't."

And finally:

> **TM:** "But I'm saying that what's actually happening in South Africa would not support these reports. I'm sure there's a misperception of what is happening in South Africa."[51]

An important critique from many public health activists is that Mbeki's unorthodox approach to AIDS, while perhaps not "untrue," had the effect of undermining South Africa's anti-AIDS campaign. His questioning of the central role of the virus, so the argument goes, relieves people from the responsibility of avoiding that virus. Other than using anecdotal stories, it would of course be difficult to demonstrate what might have happened if Mbeki had been more "conventional". An equally important and unanswerable (and usually unasked) question would be how events might have unfolded differently if the mainstream media had taken an approach more like the African media, and Mbeki had freer reign to develop his views.

Underneath the critique of Mbeki, however, is an uncomfortable assumption—uncomfortable to those who believe in true community-based (or nation-based) activity. The assumption is that there is a well-accepted approach to controlling AIDS—safe sex, condoms and anti-retroviral drugs—which, though it was first articulated in the West, is universal. This is an example of a more general assumption that many professionals hold: that approaches to economic, social, and health problems developed in international academic centers (often dominated by Western thinking) are universally applicable. The assumption is so deep that it is rarely named, even by African scholars who study in Western universities. It is an assumption that Mbeki confronted head-on.

"Africa can solve its own health problems," says Dr. Daniel J. Ncayiyana, editor of the *South African Medical Journal,* but finds this difficult in the context of "the global proselytizing of first world values that are detrimental to Africa."[52] Can the rest of the world listen long enough to realize that Western solutions may not necessarily be African solutions?

Antiretroviral Drug Treatment Policy

For some people involved with AIDS care in Africa, all these debates have been superseded by what they feel is the single remaining question facing us: how do we institute and sustain antiretroviral drug treatment in Africa? This question has gained importance since the three drug combination called HAART – Highly Active AntiRetroviral Therapy – has been shown to in fact be highly active in suppressing the HIV virus in AIDS patients. For these drug treatment activists, the importance of the Mbeki story is mostly in how Mbeki's views would enhance or inhibit treatment programs. Indeed, the recent, more widespread use of anti-retroviral drugs in Africa will certainly change the way that AIDS is debated, and for some in Africa the use of these drugs will change their lives.

Once again, it is crucial to get a wider view of how Africans living and working in Africa approach drug treatment. Many express caution, even orthodox doctors with no questions about the viral cause of AIDS. Listen again to Dr. Daniel Ncayiyana, whose article "Antiretroviral therapy cannot be South Africa's first priority" was published in the *Canadian Medical Association Journal* on June 26, 2001: He begins with an honest assessment of the problem:

> The [South African] government is regularly castigated for lacking a coherent strategy to deal with the pandemic, and efforts at implementing a consistent AIDS policy have been hobbled by a breakdown of trust and cooperation both within government and between government and nongovernmental organizations. Certainly, President Thabo Mbeki's flirtation with dissident views that deny the role of HIV in the causation of AIDS has only served to deepen the rift and to undermine the Minister of Health, whose policies and strategies are predicated on orthodox views of the syndrome.

He continued:

> Much of the criticism of the government has focused on its perceived ambivalence toward antiretroviral therapy (ART).... However, it has quite correctly been cautious about committing itself to mass prophylaxis against MTCT [mother-to-child transmission], ART, and other treatment programs, for a number of reasons.

He listed four - cost, inadequate infrastructure, lack of "capacity to counsel and test all pregnant women," and realization that "whereas ART will help alleviate suffering, it will not help to contain the scourge," and that a "disproportionate emphasis on ART in public debates could result in complacency and a false perception that there is a panacea for HIV and AIDS."

He then recognized that HIV/AIDS drugs would soon be more readily available in South Africa. But his conclusion lacked the optimism we often hear about ART:

However, in so far as ART is concerned, it may turn out to be a pyrrhic victory for the majority of AIDS sufferers in rural and periurban settlements who depend on public health facilities for their care, because the government is unlikely to be able to afford the infrastructure that is necessary for a successful universal ART program. The government is more likely to choose to devote its limited HIV/AIDS resources to programs that hold the promise of putting an end to the epidemic, which is indeed a wiser choice.[53]

Admittedly these sentiments predate the dramatic fall in ARV drug prices, as well as the increased international attention and funding for ARV programs in Africa. But drug cost was only one of Ncayiyana's concerns. He was also concerned about infrastructure and about the contribution of ARVs to "containing the scourge". He was not against ARVs as a response to AIDS; instead he was urging caution in the rush to embrace ARV programs without considering all of the implications and costs.

Is it possible to consider Ncayiyana's concerns and still propose a viable nation-wide ARV program in South Africa? There are several pilot programs in Africa with excellent results;[54] a similar program in Haiti proposes itself as a model, or standard even, of what can be done in resource-poor settings.[55] But these are small programs, run by committed people and well-funded from outside their countries. As important as this experience is, there is a major leap involved in taking these kinds of projects to scale nationally. Can pilot projects like these provide a standard for national ARV treatment programs?

Possibly – but there is another standard, another reference point for African governments. The same recent *New England Journal of Medicine* article we referred to in the Prologue, critical of the South African government's approach to AIDS, continues:

It is paradoxical that although the president, the minister of health, and others in the government have long publicly denied the link between HIV and AIDS and failed to provide high-profile leadership on this issue, the Ministry of Health has quietly formulated a comprehensive national strategic plan for HIV and AIDS that includes such vital components as education, programs for the modification of sexual behavior, and treatment of opportunistic infections.[56]

The paradox disappears if, as we have seen, the government did not deny the link between HIV and AIDS.

Could this "comprehensive national strategic plan" developed in Africa by Africans prove to be a standard for other national ARV programs? Though it is too early to tell, let us hear what Dr. Manto Tshabalala-Msimang, Health Minister of South Africa, says about the South African standard. We need to hear more completely what she says, because the press mostly ridicules her for advising people to eat garlic and African potatoes to boost their immune systems.

In January, 2003, she explained the foundation of the South African program:

> We are of the view that good nutrition has a critical role to play in the management of debilitating diseases including HIV and AIDS. There is a need to ensure that we strengthen our nutrition and health promotion programs to ensure that people know what food is good for their health. Good nutrition is critical and forms a basis for success of any medical intervention against diseases including AIDS related treatment.
>
> Clearly the challenges around food security in the region need to be addressed if we are to be successful in our endeavor to promote healthy diet and lifestyle in the region...[57]

Then in November, 2003, commenting on her department's "Operational Plan for Comprehensive Care and Treatment of People Living With HIV and Aids", which included treatment with ARVs for all who need them, she said this:

To deliver this kind of care across the country, with equitable access to all, will require a major effort to upgrade our national healthcare system. This includes the recruitment of thousands of health professionals and a very large training program to ensure that nurses, doctors, laboratory technicians, counselors and other health workers have the knowledge and the skills to ensure safe, ethical and effective use of medicines.

Built into the implementation of this program will be a massive public education campaign so that patients will know what is expected of them. This will include the provision of all the necessary information about benefits as well as dangers of usage of ARVs, to allow patients to make an informed choice.

Over half of the total budget that will be spent over the next five years in implementing this program will go to upgrading health infrastructure, emphasizing prevention, and promoting healthy lifestyles. As such, the implementation of this plan will benefit the health system as a whole.[58]

Indeed, the plan she referred to proposed only 14% of the 2003-04 AIDS treatment budget going to antiretroviral drugs, and the rest to upgrading the healthcare infrastructure. The amount proposed for drugs rises each year, and by the fifth year, 2007-08, it would account for 37%.[59] What South Africa seems to be planning for is a "new paradigm for public health" which Dr. Joia Mukherjee of Partners in Health explains: "What has succeeded before in public health are answers that are fairly straightforward and one-shot, like vaccination..." However, she continues, treating AIDS "looks at treatment of a complicated medical disease with a complicated treatment regimen on a public health scale.... We're talking about the public health treatment of a chronic condition."[60] Often, in successful pilot programs, this has involved supervised or "directly observed treatment" (DOT). While this kind of supervision is clearly more expensive than merely making drugs available, it is as important as sterile technique is in surgery: ignoring it can have disastrous consequences. It should be no surprise that only one-third of South Africa's five year budget is intended for antiretroviral drugs.

Two months before announcing the South African plan, Tshabalala-Msimang had summarized the South African approach, beginning with a quote from the new Director General of the WHO:

> The Director General of WHO, Dr Jong-Wook Lee said: "If all the money and drugs were available today, that will not solve our problem because they will not be delivered. There are simply not enough doctors, nurses and infrastructure. It is very misleading [to say] that it is a lack of drugs that is making this crisis worse."
>
> We are already facing a specter of multi-drug resistance in TB and chloroquine-resistant malaria. A robust system for monitoring and evaluation of antiretrovirals is necessary so that we do not face a greater problem of drug resistance as we scale up our response to HIV and AIDS as well.
>
> Also critical was the acknowledgment of the conditions of poverty and malnutrition that make our populations more vulnerable to HIV and other infections and cause them to succumb easily to AIDS and TB. Issues of food insecurity, malnutrition and underdevelopment remain a priority and we decided to lobby for nutritional support and intensify our efforts towards poverty alleviation. Socio-economic development is critical in pulling our populations out of the conditions of poverty and disease...[61]

This is the South African standard for ARV treatment: the government is clearly not opposed to drugs. But South Africa understands what is involved in beginning an ARV program. And if they, with one of the better developed health systems on the continent, feel that 86% of the first year's budget needs to go to preparing the system to administer the drugs, what about the rest of Africa? In the African context, perhaps the South African plan would be a good standard, a good reference point for all of Africa.

References

[1] *http://www.whitehouse.gov/news/releases/2003/05/20030527-7.html*

[2] **Green, Edward (2003)**, "A Plan as Simple as ABC", *New York Times* Opinion, March 1.

[3] *www.anc.org.za/ancdocs/history/mbeki/1998/tm1009.htm*

[4] **Underhill, Glynnis (1998)**, "Health Minister Zuma Faces Court Action on AZT" and "Government's Decision to Withdraw Drugs Angers Those with AIDS", both Global News Wire, Nov.1.

[5] *www.gov.za/search97cgi/s97_cgi?action+View?VdkVgwKey+%2E%2E%2Fd ata%2...*

[6] **South African Press Association (1999)**, Cape AIDS Gathering Attacks Mbeki on AZT", Dec.1; **O'Malley, Padraig (2004)**, "A South African 'genocide' in AIDS policies," *Boston Globe* Op-Ed, April 13.

[7] **Mugambi, J.N.K (1989)**, *Christianity and African Culture* (Nairobi, Acton Publishers), p. 190.

[8] **Swarns, Rachel (2000)**, *The New York Times*, March 19.

[9] **Baleta, Adele (2000)**, "Questioning of HIV theory of AIDS causes dismay in South Africa," *The Lancet*, vol 355, no 9210, April 1.

[10] **Sidley, Pat (2000)**, "Clouding the AIDS issue", *BMJ*, 320:1016, April 8.

[11] *www.sumeria.net/aids/mbekiltr.html*

[12] **Gellman, Barton (2000)**, "S. African President Escalates AIDS Feud; Mbeki Challenges Western Remedies", *The Washington Post*, April 19.

[13] **Bayer, Ronald and Susser, Mervyn (2000)**, "In South Africa, AIDS and a Dangerous Denial", *The Washington Post*, April 20

[14] **Orina, Eric (2000)**, "Mbeki's Letter on AIDS Made the West See Red," *The Nation* (Kenya), April 26.

[15] This, and other quotes in this section, are from **Louise Lander (1978)**, *Defective Medicine: Risk, Anger, and the Malpractice Crisis,* (New York, Farrar, Straus, and Giroux), p. 79-81, 84, and 89. Her quote here is from **Rene Dubos (1959)**, *Mirage of Health: Utopias, Progress, and Biological Change,* (New York, Harper and Row,) p. 131.

[16] **Geiger, H. Jack (1975)**, "The Illusion of Change," *Social Policy* 6(3):30-35 at p. 33 (Nov-Dec, 1975), quoted in **Lander (1978)**, *Defective Medicine,* p.83.

[17] **Dubos (1959)**, *Mirage of Health,* (New York, Harper and Row) p. 118.

[18] For example, **Ivan Illich (1976)**, *Medical Nemesis: The Expropriation of Health* (London, BMJ Publishing); **Louise Lander (1978)**, *Defective Medicine;* **Thomas McKeown (1979)**, *The Role of Medicine: Dream, Mirage, or Nemesis* (Princeton, Princeton University Press); **Ian Kennedy (1981)**, *The Unmasking of Medicine* (London, Granada Publishers); and **Stephen Kunitz (1983)**, *Disease Change and the Role of Medicine: The Navajo Experience* (Berkeley, University of California Press).

[19] **Kunitz, Stephen (1983)**, *Disease Change and the Role of Medicine* (Berkeley, University of California Press) p. 186.

[20] **Mbeki, Thabo**, "Prologue" to *African Renaissance,* edited by M W Makgoba **(1999)** (Cape Town, Mafube Publishing and Tafelberg Publishing), p. xxi.

[21] **The NewsHour with Jim Lehrer, Monday, (2000)** May 22, Transcript #6733.

[22] *www.anc.org.za/ancdocs/history/mbeki/2000/tm0506.html*

[23] **Conlan, Mark (2000a)**, "South African AIDS Debate Panel Holds First Meeting in May", interview with Peter Duesberg and David Rasnick,

Rethinking AIDS, vol 8, no.6, June.

[24] **Scondras, David (2000),** "The HIV Controversy: Face-off with the Flat-earthers", October. *www.poz.com/archive/October00/features/hivcontroversy.html*

[25] **Conlan, Mark,** *op.cit,* **2000a.**

[26] "All the President's Scientists: Diary of a Round-earther", *Mail and Guardian* (South Africa), 08 09 2000.

[27] **Conlan, Mark (2000b),** "South African AIDS Reappraisal Panel Completes Second Meeting", interview with David Rasnick and Charles Geshekter, *Rethinking AIDS,* vol 8, no.8, August.

[28] **Christie, Huw (2000),** "Suspend All HIV Testing Mbeki Expert Panel Recommends", *New African,* September.

[29] **Schoofs, Mark (2000),** "Debating the Obvious: Inside the South African Government's Controversial AIDS Panel", *The Village Voice,* July 5-11.

[30] "The Durban Declaration," *Nature* 406, 15-16 (July 6, 2000).

[31] **Prabhakara, MS (2000),** "S Africa still harbors Eurocentric mindset," *The Hindu* (India), October 8.

[32] *www.anc.org.za/ancdocs/history/mbeki/2000/tm0709.html*

[33] **Farmer, Paul (2001),** "Health Hazard / AIDS", New *Internationalist,* 331, Jan/Feb.

[34] "Mbeki's AIDS Speech Disappoints", UN Integrated Regional Information Network, July 10, 2000.

[35] **Horton, Richard (2000),** "Mbeki Defiant About South African HIV/AIDS Strategy," *Lancet* 356 (9225): 225, July 15.

[36] **Brown, D and Jeter, J (2000),** "Hundreds Walk Out On Mbeki", *Washington Post,* July 10.

[37] **Barber, Simon (2000)**, "Lazy journalist virus causes herd-like motion in Durban," *Business Day*, July 12.

[38] **Brown, D and Jeter, J,** *op. cit.*, **2000.**

[39] **Cohen, Jon (2000)**, "Companies, Donors Pledge to Close Gap in AIDS Treatment," *Science Magazine*, 289 (5478): 368, July 21.

[40] **Kalyegira, Timothy (2000)**, "South Africa calls for African approach to AIDS," UPI International, July 2.

[41] "South Africa: Controversy at AIDS Forum," *The Dispatch* (Accra), July 15, 2000.

[42] **Wendo, Charles (2000)**, "Health Minister Corrects Mbeki's AIDS Claim," *New Vision*, July 19.

[43] **Mulugeta, Allehone (2000)**, "Africa and the AIDS Debate," *Addis Tribune*, August 11.

[44] **Mwale, Sam (2000)**, "Was Bad Science the Source of Aids in Africa?", *The East African* (Nairobi), September 28.

[45] **Ayodele, Funmi (2000)**, "South African Doctors Fault Mbeki's View on HIV/AIDS," *This Day* (Lagos), October 5.

[46] "Kenyan Doctor Defends Mbeki on AIDS," *Panafrican News Agency*, December 2, 2000.

[47] "Time Europe Interview with President Mbeki", *Time Europe*, vol 156, no 11, Sept.11, 2000.

[48] *http://www.gcis.gov.za/media/releases/000914.htm*

[49] Interview with Debra Patta, April 24, 2001 on eTV "On The Record", recorded in *New African*, June, 2001.

[50] **Barrell, Howard (2000)**, "Mbeki fingers the CIA in Aids conspiracy" and "What the president said...," *Mail and Guardian*, October 6.

[51] **Sebastian, Tim (2001),** "Interview with President Thabo Mbeki," *BBC World's Hard Talk,* Aug. 6, *http://www.virusmyth.net/aids/news/tsinterviewtm.htm.*

[52] **Ncayiyana, Daniel (2002),** "Africa can solve its own health problems," *BMJ,* 324:688-9, March 23.

[53] **Ncayiyana, Daniel (2001),** "Antiretroviral therapy cannot be South Africa's first priority," *CMAJ,* June 26.

[54] **Oransky, Ivan (2003),** "African patients adhere well to anti-HIV regimens," *Lancet* v. 362 n 9387 13.

[55] **Farmer, Paul et al (2001),** "Community-based approaches to HIV treatment in resource-poor settings," *Lancet* v. 358 n. 9279, p 404-409, 4 August.

[56] **Benatar, Solomon (2004),** "Health Care Reform and the Crisis of HIV and AIDS in South Africa," *NEJM* 351:1, p. 86-7.

[57] **Tshabalala-Msimang, Manto (2003a),** "SADC Consultative Meeting on Nutrition and HIV/AIDS," *www.doh.gov.za/docs/pr/2003/pr0121.html*

[58] **Tshabalala-Msimang, Manto,** "Statement of Cabinet on a Plan for Comprehensive Treatment and Care for HIV and AIDS in South Africa," *www.gov.za/search97cgi/s97_cgi?action=View&VdkVgwKey=%2E%2E%2Fd ata%2...*

[59] "Cabinet=s Decision On The Operational Plan For Comprehensive Care And Treatment Of People Living With Hiv And Aids," *www.doh.gov.za/docs/pr/2003/pr1119.html*

[60] Quoted in **D'Adesky, Anne-Christine (2004),** *Moving Mountains: The Race to Treat Global AIDS* (London, Verso), p. 107.

[61] **Tshabalala-Msimang, Manto (2003b),** "Health: African Work Together to Meet Health Challenges," *ANC Today,* Vol 3, No 36, 12-18 September, *http://www.anc.org.za/ancdocs/anctoday/2003/text/at36.txt*

4

Nkozi:
The Maturation of the African AIDS Discourse

To many, the July 2000 International AIDS Conference in Durban, South Africa, was a landmark meeting. For those who follow the conventional Western approach, it was the place where Mbeki failed to make clear that HIV causes AIDS, and the occasion for the Durban Declaration which did make that clear. For Western dissidents, it was the place where Mbeki stood up to the orthodox Westerners and, for a while at least, fueled the dissident case that HIV does *not* cause AIDS. The theme was "Break the Silence", and for nearly everyone, some sort of silence was broken. Everyone, that is, except those Africans who felt that the microbial etiology was not the most pressing question—and Mbeki was ironically one of them.

Less than two months later there was another AIDS conference in Africa that did break that silence, that did give voice to some distinctly African views. It was not the only time that silence was broken—we already noted that Baffour Ankomah, in all his articles for the *New African*, did not declare himself for or against a viral etiology of AIDS —but this other conference deserves a closer look because of its context following the Durban meeting. It was in Nkozi, Uganda—and the two conferences were as different as their venues.

Durban is a big, modern, busy city: pleasant, efficient, and cosmopolitan. Nkozi is a small, rural Ugandan village an hour away from Kampala. In Durban's central park there is now a huge memorial to Gugu Dlamini, the woman who was lynched and beaten to death in 1998 when she declared publicly that she was HIV positive. On the road from Kampala to Nkozi the AIDS education billboards are faded; the newer slicker ones advertise cell phones and Pepsi, and proclaim that "Coffee Eradicates Poverty". Durban has an International Convention Centre which hosted the 10,000 people attending the XIII International AIDS Conference;

Nkozi has motor-scooter taxis from the main road to the small Catholic university where the other conference was held.

It was almost not held. Some of the same dissidents who were so proud of Mbeki had helped to organize this smaller conference at Uganda Martyrs University around the theme "Making Sense: Alternative Views on the Origins and Causes of AIDS in Africa". Among the organizers was Rosalind Harrison-Chirimuuta, who a decade earlier with her husband Richard had written *AIDS, Africa and Racism*.[1] This was one of the earlier works questioning the scientific dogma surrounding the African origins of HIV—but not, interestingly, its existence. However, because their work dissented from dogma, they were grouped with other dissidents. The Ugandan government got nervous, warning "that if the conference focused on conflicting views and myths, it would undermine the gains already made in Uganda in the struggle against HIV/AIDS."[2] Government officials postponed the opening of the conference, met with the conference organizers, and engineered a compromise: if the organizers would "downgrade the conference to an academic discourse and not release any material on the conference proceedings to the press," the government would not "deploy police to block the conference."[3]

The conference opened a day late, attended by dozens, not thousands. The compromise was an interesting one. The title and theme of the conference changed to "A Holistic Approach: An International Conference on the Fight Against AIDS in Africa," but the contents seemed to follow the original plan. The government, for its part, convened a parallel meeting in Kampala, attended by Luc Montaigner, the co-discoverer of the AIDS virus[4]—apparently attempting to lure media attention away from the "alternative" or "holistic" conference.[5]

At first glance, it looks like this conference was simply a dissident event on African soil, with the usual dissident issues being raised. Dr. Kevin Corbett from the UK, one of the organizers of the conference, raised questions about the accuracy of the diagnostic tests on which so many of the statistics are based. Dr. Rheeta Moran, also from the UK, said, "Drugs that are not working in the West are being dumped in Africa." And Prof. Sam Mhlongo, one of the South Africans who sat on President Mbeki's Panel, said the HIV virus had not even been isolated yet. It was perhaps no surprise that the recommendations at the end of the conference included, among others:

- that Africa should suspend all HIV/Aids testing until the virus has been isolated;
- African countries suspend use of anti-retrovirals for treatment of Aids until the virus is isolated;
- that search for an HIV vaccine be suspended and resources re-routed to more pressing health problems;...
- all adverts relating to HIV/Aids be banned.[6]

That, at least, is the way the story was reported in an East African newspaper.

The official report and recommendations published later[7] by the conference conveners, however, were more nuanced. Their first recommendation, of seven, was: "Our countries should ensure that there is adequate provision of health, educational, and social care resources. AIDS should be discussed and addressed in conjunction with the issues of human welfare, need and development." Regarding vaccine research, it said, "Current research on developing a vaccine for HIV must be refocused and reviewed in the light of the questions and doubts about the isolation of HIV." This wasn't exactly the sound-bite reported above.

Likewise, the recommendation regarding testing was more complex. "HIV testing should be suspended. If testing for HIV is undertaken there should be full information about the non-specificity of the tests and pre-and post-test counseling should be provided."

Regarding treatment, the official conference recommendation was more limited than was reported in the media: "Without incontrovertible evidence of their benefit, policies of antiretroviral treatment *for pregnant women and their infants* and the substitution of formula for breast milk should not be implemented." Their comment about treatment of AIDS with ARVs was, "The treatment *emphasis* for AIDS must be shifted from the provision of expensive and toxic antiretroviral drugs to tried and tested interventions." [italics mine].

Finally, the media recommendation was much less controversial than the newspaper reported: "The media in Africa should investigate thoroughly and report responsibly on all issues around AIDS/HIV without relying on medico-pharmaceutical press releases or reports from Western countries." This need for "reporting responsibly" was ironically demonstrated by the differences just outlined between the conference documents and the media reports.

Even more ironic, perhaps, was the fate of the two public outlets which carried these official recommendations. I downloaded them from a website devoted specifically to the conference, a website which is now apparently non-functional. I also found them in the magazine *Continuum*, published in Britain during the 1990s and focusing on alternative or dissident views of several health issues, especially AIDS. The issue carrying these recommendations had several other comprehensive articles about the Mbeki story. The following issue the next year was their last; the magazine closed shortly after the editor, Huw Christie, died—of AIDS.[8]

The Western dissident agenda, focusing on the microbial etiology of AIDS, seems to be losing steam. If the Nkozi conference was just another opportunity for dissidents to be heard, it would have little historic importance. However, as we have already seen, the "official" recommendations were less radical, or less "dissident", than they were first reported to be. But beyond this, there were three other papers presented at the conference which take the entire discussion onto a different level. They were available, though somewhat hidden, on the now defunct conference website, and one of them was reprinted on other dissident websites. All of these papers were by African scholars, professors at Uganda universities. All of them referred favorably, if briefly, to Mbeki. And none of them entertained the question of the viral cause of AIDS, nor the merits of HIV testing, nor the major debates over drug therapy. In some very profound ways they—not the Western dissidents—picked up where Mbeki left off.

95

INTERLUDE II—Miasma and Contagion

Before looking in detail at what these scholars have contributed to an African understanding of AIDS, it will be necessary to take another "interlude", similar to, and built on, the one in the middle of the Mbeki story. In that interlude we reviewed the role of drugs in the Western biomedical model. Drugs are chosen based on their ability to inhibit the specific agent causing the disease. That theory, of course, assumes there is a specific agent responsible for every disease: "the doctrine of specific etiology, or causation"—an expansion of the germ theory of disease.

The critique we noted then was that this approach can be reductionistic, ignoring social or environmental causes of disease, as well as ignoring the treatment approaches that those causes might suggest. It would at first seem that this critique is unfair: some common diseases in the West, such as coronary artery disease, do not fit this pattern of "specific etiology", and we recognize multiple factors leading to them. We therefore employ multiple approaches in treating them: smoking cessation, diet counseling, and exercise are at least as important as drugs. Yet while followers of the biomedical model would agree with this, there is still a specific etiology—or specific etiologies—assumption: we are still looking for the specific factors (cholesterol level, blood pressure, etc.) that these interventions modify. The idea is that modifying (or destroying) each factor helps to treat or prevent the disease. The whole is simply the sum of the parts—the parts that we can identify.

Medicine has not always been so focused. Throughout history people have debated where diseases came from (especially the most common diseases, which were infectious), and by the Nineteenth Century there were two major theories: miasma and contagion. Miasma said that certain *places* had diseases, caused by the surrounding, often filthy, atmosphere. Contagion said that certain *people* had diseases, and could spread them to other people by direct contact. Some diseases, such as malaria, seemed best explained by miasma; others, such as smallpox, fit better with contagion. Miasma followers argued that to prevent disease, the places needed to be cleaned up; contagionists said that to prevent disease spreading, the people with it needed to be quarantined. Interestingly, before the discovery of bacteria and parasites as the causes of infectious diseases, both approaches were successful in containing the spread of these diseases.

However, with the advent of bacteriology in the late Nineteenth Century, it appeared that the contagion party had won. There was now proof that all infectious diseases were caused by specific living things—germs—that grew in people and could spread to other people. It may have been insects that spread some of the diseases (like malaria), while direct contact spread others (like smallpox). Nevertheless, it was the germs in the people that were causing the disease—and subsequently science found drugs that would kill those germs. Miasma, it would appear, belonged with humoral theories of disease and bloodletting: in history books.

However, it may be that miasma was relegated to the history books too soon. Contagion explained very well *how* a person became ill, but not *why*—why that particular person at that time. Miasma was admittedly vague on *how*, but successfully predicted at least where people would get ill—where the filthy miasma was. Contagion granted that mosquitoes bred in swamps, rats fed on refuse piles, and polluted water supplies contained pathogenic bacteria, and had no objection to them being cleaned up. But the question of why one person became infected and another didn't was left unanswered by those who looked only at germs. Or almost unanswered. Pasteur, one of the fathers of the contagion theory, reportedly said on his death bed "the microbe is nothing, the terrain is everything."

But his dying passion did not reverse the focus on the microbes. As science developed more and more techniques—and especially drugs—to prevent and kill germs, attention on the polluted environment has decreased. Now we prevent malaria with prophylactic drugs and mosquito nets, we prevent measles with immunization, we recommend hand washing and boiling water to prevent cholera—and we recommend condoms and post-exposure prophylaxis to prevent AIDS. Medicine has no objection to draining swamps or reducing poverty or sexual continence, but—and here is the key—these are not medicine. HIV/AIDS is a disease, and so (we believe but rarely state) AIDS belongs primarily to medicine.

It is this—that AIDS is a disease and belongs to medicine—that fuels the way we research and report on and try to control AIDS. And as we have seen, medicine carries certain unstated assumptions—such as the doctrine of specific etiology, and the preference for contagion rather than miasma. Yet as we showed above, contagion won over miasma, not because miasma was proven wrong, but simply because contagion was proven right. All of the truths of miasma—that certain places contained something that led to disease, and that cleaning up that something prevented the disease—were still true, but now had no legitimate theory within medicine to carry them. Some of these miasma perspectives shifted out of medicine into the social sciences and urban planning and public health—disciplines that always play second fiddle to the more dramatic and increasingly "successful" contagion-based medicine. But some of the ideas of miasma remain unexamined in our subconscious, and creep up equally unexamined as theories of, for example, why Africans get AIDS.

Nkozi

Nduhukhire-Owa-Mataze calls these theories "suspicious conceptual frameworks".[9] He is one of the three Ugandan scholars who presented papers at the Nkozi conference. By addressing conceptual frameworks he was broadening the discussion of what causes AIDS beyond the simple matter of microbes. Contagion-based science could explain why an individual African was ill from AIDS, but could not explain why far more Africans than Americans had AIDS, even though the disease appeared in both places at about the same time. It began to seem that there was some "miasma" in Africa responsible for the epidemic. But since we don't believe in miasma any more, and since the truths of miasma don't have a scientific home, several miasma-like theories began to occur. It is these theories that Owa-Mataze called "suspicious".

He began by asking, "Are contemporary theoretical frameworks employed in analyzing HIV/AIDS 'objective'?" It is a stark question for scientists. Owa-Mataze looks at several explanations for why there is more AIDS in Africa. Some have suggested that AIDS originated and flourishes in Africa because of poverty—but then they describe that poverty as the scarcity of Western goods and the lack of Western social and political values. In this "black peril" view, Africa has AIDS because it is not Western—a thesis Owa-Mataze naturally rejects.

Only slightly more "scientific" is the "distinct sexuality" perspective, a view suggesting Africans are a "people whose sexuality is inherently permissive." Owa-Mataze also rejects this, pointing out that if anything Western values have contributed to the distortion of African sexual values. "Like all the other narrow and racially-driven world-views that 'scientists' have taken aboard without any serious questioning, the theses view Africans as totally irresponsible and barbaric, particularly in the art of sex. They must, consequently, be forced to adopt 'other' peoples' social values"—including the use of condoms. Once again, Owa-Mataze sees Westerners using their values as the standards by which to examine and evaluate Africans.

A third problematic framework he sees is the focus on "high-risk occupational groups"—prostitutes, truck drivers, bar maids, itinerant workers, and those who work in tourism and entertainment. While AIDS may be more common among them—and as a result, international labor groups have outlawed discrimination against them—Owa-Mataze notes that these same labor groups have been too narrow in their approach. They have not explored "the relationship between the market and money-centered activities, the changing expectations and the erosion of African sexual values." In addition, while opposing stigmatization of workers, they have not opposed "the stigmatization and discrimination of Africa and its people."

Overall, Owa-Mataze suggests, these suspicious frameworks look for the miasma within Africa and Africans, but fail to see outside forces that have made Africans susceptible to AIDS. "What about the centuries of poverty, exploitation, brutalities, immoralities and the de-humanization that colonialism and post-colonial wards and distortions have unleashed on the people of the area?" he asks. And then, more directly, "What of the poverty of borrowed Western medical frameworks that use the region largely as a market for pharmaceutical products and experimental centers for drugs that are not contextualized in regard to African conditions?"

Owa-Mataze does not enter the debate about whether or not HIV causes AIDS. His concern is with miasma, not contagion; but first with exposing some inadequate miasmic theories from the West. He realizes that Mbeki too was not primarily concerned with viral questions: Mbeki, in questioning the scientific claims and calling "for more critical analyses on the real causes of AIDS," had highlighted the link between AIDS and massive poverty. But "in the eyes of neo-liberal scientists and scholars, [he] had committed a more serious crime by linking HIV and AIDS with the current globalization and the accompanying massive exploitation and marginalization of the continent." If this was truly his more serious crime, even the scientists knew that Mbeki was not discussing contagion, but miasma — only his approach to miasma was different from theirs: different and threatening.

Another speaker, Peter Kanyandago, one of the co-organizers of the conference, reinforced Mbeki's and Owa-Mataze's contentions in his paper.[10] "Africa is not poor, but impoverished," he said — and gave this evidence: "every day, $60m is transferred from the poorest countries to the richest in debt repayments." While this phenomenon of cash transfer may be recent, Kanyandago shows that the "process of negation and exploitation" has been ongoing, resulting in the myths of black sexuality mentioned above, as well as recent references to Africa as the "hopeless continent". The most fundamental negation is that "the humanity of the African has been questioned." All of this says that "Africans are underdeveloped and poor, and therefore unable to solve their problems, including that of AIDS."

Kanyandago, of course, does not believe this: "In order to be able to solve their problems, including that of immune deficiency in general and of AIDS in particular, Africa must start by retrieving and defending their cultural identity, by regaining control over their resources, and by instituting processes for reconciliation and healing." By speaking of immune deficiency in general and AIDS in particular in the same sentence, Kanyandago has conflated miasma and contagion; while not denying the virus, he also chooses not to see viral-caused immune deficiency (AIDS) as in a totally different category from all other deficiencies of immunity.

"Mbeki's stand," he continues, "that the solution to the problem of AIDS on the continent must be an African solution, should be supported." At the beginning of his paper he gave the reason for the necessity of this affirmation of African solutions:

> Today it is taken for granted that if Africa is to find a solution to the problem of AIDS, and other problems, it must accept aid and medicine from the West. It is presumed that Africa cannot scientifically and economically manage this problem because it is poor, and therefore needs to be assisted.

Owa-Mataze was likewise concerned about this assumption, and especially about "the African leaders and a few scholars who have kept quiet in the face of increased racist conclusions.... Where in Africa are the voices in protest...?" he asks, beyond "Mbeki's lonely voice in protest." But of course he recognizes the pressure: "African leaders and scholars whose economies now depend on aid were consequently told to keep their mouths closed however much their people were abused." Likewise, most international organizations "prefer to cheer on African governments as they focus on HIV/AIDS rather than other kinds of malaise that... are as deadly if not worse than HIV/AIDS." Once again, the Western emphasis on contagion and germs overshadows any African attempts to address miasma.

To Owa-Mataze, the reasons for this imbalance are clear: HIV/AIDS has "become a new venture in reactivating private capital investments in drugs-manufacturing and research." Consequently, the suggestion by Mbeki that poverty was more important than a drug-sensitive virus was dangerous to these financial concerns: "that voice could not be allowed to influence others on the continent that is increasingly becoming a good market for HIV and AIDS drugs and condoms." Other African leaders "had to be seriously warned against questioning what the global community of capital sees as the problem to be solved by global inventions."

The third African presenter, Emmanuel Katongole, took the discussion in a different direction.[11] Until now we have been considering why Africa has more AIDS—or at least why the West thinks Africa has more AIDS, and how these theories are "suspicious" and racist. We have also heard that though the approach to African AIDS must be African, Western hegemony inhibits this. Given then that Western approaches are now preeminent in the fight against AIDS, Katongole asks how these approaches have affected Africa: "as we make particular decisions and choices ... what sort of people are we becoming?"

He begins where Owa-Mataze does, looking at Western views of Africa, agreeing that these misleading and racist approaches are suspicious frameworks. But if the frameworks are suspicious, the obvious result is that people observing these frameworks—first the scholars and intellectuals, but eventually all Africans—become suspicious of the West. He sees this suspicion increasing as a result of the AIDS epidemic and the West's narrow approach to it: "President Thabo Mbeki has rightly questioned the determination of HIV/Aids incidence in Africa which so narrowly focuses on 'viral infection' and overlooks the wider economic and political and general health conditions in Africa." Africans become suspicious when a restricted concentration on contagion crowds out any consideration of miasma.

But becoming suspicious has a cost: "…we [may] need a certain measure of suspicion as part of the practical wisdom of everyday life and survival. The challenge of course is to ensure that such suspicion is kept within moral bounds...." And this is where Katongole sees the problem in what sort of people Africans are becoming. They have not only become suspicious of the West, they have also been told by the Western approach to AIDS to become suspicious of each other.

I remember in the early 80s when, at least in Uganda, billboards warning against the spread of HIV infection carried the picture of what was obviously a married couple with their three young children, and bore the caption: 'Love Faithfully to Avoid Aids'. This recommendation was soon replaced by the Uganda Aids Commission with what was seen to be a more potent picture: two young lovers in embrace, with the caption: 'Love Carefully'. What the Uganda Aids Commission might not have realized, but what in fact it was confirming was the realization that with Aids even lovers cannot (or is it, should not) trust each other fully (love faithfully), but must learn the art of loving 'carefully', that is, suspiciously. Apparently it did not take a long time to realize that such 'careful' love involves regarding the partner as potential danger from which one had to 'protect' oneself. Thus, by mid 90s the captions had changed again, this time from 'Love Carefully' to 'Use a Condom' to Avoid Aids.

The West may have long ago adopted this mutual suspicion, but it is new to Africa: this "radical suspicion generated by Aids gnaws at the very core of our self-understanding, and thus threatens the basic trust on which our individual and societal existence is based," Katongole says.

In response to this mistrust, instead of addressing how Africans can rebuild trust, the West has promoted condoms. One of the leading brands heavily financed by Western money is even called Trust. Katongole calls this process of sidestepping the fundamental issues "condomization". "The issue of course is not whether condoms do or do not protect against the spread of AIDS.... The issue is about the sort of culture which 'condomization' promotes, and the sort of people we become as a result." Condomization becomes a "metaphor for the incursion of postmodern culture in Africa."

Some may see that incursion as an inevitable effect of globalization. Katongole, as an African, describes three fundamental problems with that incursion. He argues that condoms are, like so many other aspects of Western culture, disposable. But condomization "is not just about the convenience of disposable condoms, but more importantly it is about the popularization of a certain form of sexual activity, i.e., one detached from any serious attachment or stable commitment. In other words, condomization encourages one to view sex, and one's sex partner(s) as essentially disposable, while at the same time parading such lack of attachment as a high mark of freedom and accomplishment."

This "freedom" is the second problem with condomization, which he identified. Using a condom seems to confer immediate freedom—but of course "freedom does not come naturally, but is a result of *training* into the relevant virtues of chastity, fidelity, and self-control." That, at least, is the teaching of church and ethnic traditions. Without this training, these free people become "free-floating individuals who easily become prey to their own whimsical needs and choices."

These whimsical choices Katongole calls "nihilistic playfulness", the third problem with the incursion of postmodern culture into Africa. "One wonders, however, whether we in Africa can afford the playfulness of such 'it feels good' culture, which in the West is not only made possible by the economic infrastructure of advanced capitalism, but also masks the deep frustration and nihilism within postmodern affluence."

This of course is a stinging critique of the West itself. But Katongole's intent is to pursue what effect this condomization has within Africa. It "transforms Africans into free-floating individuals, incapable of any deep attachments, but [with] a certain superficial feeling and playfulness." When this happens,

> we lose not only the possibility of locating ourselves within any meaningful material economic practices and history, but even more crucially, we become increasingly prey to the manipulations and misrepresentations of the media and market forces.... It may not be a long shot to see a connection between this form of nihilistic playfulness and the various forms of desperate violence with many

countries in Africa. Such violence may be just an indication that the extreme form of cynicism, namely fatalism is, for many Africans, just around the corner."

When the scientists of the late 19th century discovered bacteria to be the cause of some diseases, they moved ahead the possibility for improved disease control—and they gave a boost to the theory of contagion, elbowing out miasma in the process. Focusing on bacteria and parasites was more accurate than focusing on swamps and piles of garbage. The germ could be considered and dealt with apart from its source; it had become autonomous, no longer just a vague part of the miasma. Understanding the germ autonomously had great benefit in allowing the development of methods to control and kill it. The benefit was so great, in fact, that science felt justified in eliminating the concept of miasma: piles of garbage were dangerous not because they looked bad or smelled bad, but because—*only* because—they contained germs.

A similar process has been taking place in philosophy over the last two centuries, at least in the West. People are now viewed as autonomous individuals, not merely vague parts of their families or communities. Individual autonomy has become a cornerstone value of medical ethics; people are now freed from the cultural or moral codes they cannot accept because they no longer believe in them. We have accepted the progression from "I think, therefore I am" to "I think differently from you, therefore I am different from you." The final step, which some celebrate and others bemoan, is "I think alone, therefore I am alone." Those who celebrate it have embraced playful nihilism.

Autonomous germs, autonomous people. In opting for autonomy as their basis, both medical science and ethics have made a Faustian deal. They have chosen paths that lead to apparent progress and freedom, but in doing so have stopped looking at where those germs and where those people come from. Some Africans have begun pointing out the inadequacies of this approach to AIDS in Africa. Could it be that the autonomous approach is also inadequate for treating disease in the West?

References

[1] **Chirimuuta, Richard and Chirimuuta, Rosalind (1989),** *AIDS, Africa and Racism,* (London, Free Association Books).

[2] "Dissident Indaba Brought to Heel", August 29, 2000, *www.credence.org/Eclub/Sept14th2000.htm*

[3] **Wakabi, Michael (2000),** "Uganda to Allow Conference by Dissenters on Cause of AIDS," *Business Day* (South Africa), August 29.

[4] **Harrison, Rosiland (2000),** "A Tale of Two AIDS Conferences," *New African,* December.

[5] **Wakabi,** *op.cit.* **2000.**

[6] **Kirauni, Lucy (2000),** "AIDS: Controversy Over the Disease Still Rages," *East African Standard,* September 12.

[7] **Africa AIDS website**, not currently functional *www.africanaids.org/media/nkozi.pdf.* Also published in *Continuum* (London), vol 6, no.2, October, 2000.

[8] *http://www.virusmyth.net/aids/data/mbobituaryhc.htm*

[9] **Owa-Mataze, Nduhukhire (2000),** "HIV, AIDS, and The New Xenophobia: Save Africa from Stigmatization," paper presented at the Nkozi Conference, 28 Aug- 1 Sept., downloaded from *www.africanaids.org/media/mataze.pdf*

[10] **Kanyandago, Peter (2000),** "AIDS in Africa: Anthropological and Ethical Questions," presented at Nkozi 28 Aug- 1 Sept., downloaded from *www.africanaids.org/media/kanyand.pdf.*

[11] **Katongole, Emmanuel (2000a),** "AIDS, Ethics and Society in Africa: Exploring the Limits of an Ethics of Suspicion," presented at Nkozi 28 Aug—1 Sept., 2000, downloaded from *www.africanaids.org/media/katongol.pdf.* Also available at *http://aidsmyth.addr.com/articles/katongole.htm.* The ideas in this presentation are also available in two published articles by Katongole: "Postmodern

Illusions and the Challenges of African Theology: The Ecclesial Tactics of Resistance," *Modern Theology* 16:2 April 2000, p. 237-254; and "Christian Ethics and AIDS in Africa Today: Exploring the Limits of a Culture of Suspicion and Despair," *Missionalia* 29:2, August 2001, p.144-160.

5

Philosophy, Theology, and Gender:
The Mainstream Foundations of the African
AIDS Discourse

Until now, we have seen that the distinctly African discourse of AIDS draws partly from the Western dissident discourse. Some of the early sources used by the *New African* were dissidents, and some of those same dissidents organized the Nkozi conference. However, as we have tried to show, this was more of an overlap than a cause-and-effect. The fundamental dissident questions were about microbial etiology; the fundamental African questions concerned the overall approaches to AIDS being developed in the West. It is an understandable error to equate the two: the tiny Western dissident discourse has gotten more media attention in the West than the widespread grass-roots African attitudes. Where those African attitudes overlap with the Western dissidents, it is tempting—though inaccurate—to simply call the Africans dissidents, as we have seen with Mbeki.

But what do we do with African attitudes different from our own that do *not* overlap with Western dissidents? Perhaps we aren't aware of them since the media, uncertain about what to do with them, ignores them. Or perhaps we do notice attitudes that do not fit into our Western categories, and find ourselves concluding that Africa is simply "uncivilized". It is difficult for us in the West—we who analyze other cultures—to see our own ethnocentrism.

Consider the matter of ARVs to treat AIDS. The loudest voices I have heard clamoring for immediate access to ARVs in Africa are Western voices, together with the activists in South Africa. As we will see in the next chapter, some of the media reports from east Africa downplayed the importance of drug therapy when reporting on the September, 2003 AIDS conference in Nairobi. After that conference, as I traveled through eastern and southern Africa asking people what they thought of Western approaches, especially condoms and drugs, I found support for them—but only muted support. Few people felt that they had no role, but equally few felt they were pivotal. These are not "dissident" ideas, but neither do they line up with the standard Western approaches. When we realize there is a difference in approaches, how can we explain it?

Since AIDS is a disease, we assume that the disciplines that study diseases, the medical sciences, will inform us adequately. Further, since we assume that these "hard" sciences are the same world-wide, we don't feel it necessary to know the race or ethnicity of the researcher; science is science, regardless of who does it or where it's done. Science tells us that AIDS is caused by a virus, and ARVs inhibit that virus. Surely there's not an "African science" that comes to different conclusions?

No, there isn't. The "distinctly African" discourse that we have been trying to describe is not in microbiology or pharmacology. These sciences and their methods are merely techniques—very powerful techniques to be sure, but still techniques. They do not contain tools to help answer profound personal, social, economic, and metaphysical questions. They tell us the mechanics of AIDS infection, but not why it exists; they provide us with complex expensive means of inhibiting the growth of the virus after a person already has it, but cannot address the question of whether and when to use these means.

Many Westerners, of course, know this—those Westerners involved in the social sciences and humanities. Fortunately, Africans have also contributed to these "mainstream" disciplines from their distinctly African perspectives, and in these disciplines the conclusions, and even approaches, of Africans sometimes differ from their Western counterparts. In this chapter we will try to locate this African thinking in its larger philosophical framework, namely postmodernism. Following this we will consider how African theology has approached AIDS, and then survey some African gender perspectives.

Philosophy

From the perspective of medical science and the media, AIDS was at first a disease of gay men in the United States. Before long it was described in other "high risk groups", so that in the early 1980s it was the "4H" disease – found in homosexuals, Haitians, heroin users, and hemophiliacs. Since these first reports of AIDS were in people other than "normal" Americans – that is, white, heterosexual, middle class, otherwise healthy Americans – the medical community focused on what was different about those groups in order to uncover the cause. A correspondingly early response by the public at large was to blame those groups – a response several writers identified and critiqued.[1]

Clearly the largest and most articulate group in the US was the homosexuals, and their response was not just to the disease, but also to the way they saw it being handled by the medical community and the media. Their response in this atmosphere of blame was to focus instead on what treatment options were available, and how vigorously they were being developed. It was, in other words, an activist response. And it was eventually heard, in America at least, for two very different reasons. First, gay men were dying, and the pathology underlying those deaths was a major challenge to medical science. But beyond this, the gay movement's self-description came at a time in the West when intellectuals at least were willing to take "otherness" seriously. This is the postmodern celebration of difference.

Homosexuals were *different*, Haitians were *different* – and Africans, who now allegedly carry the largest AIDS burden, were also different. It is understandable then that the response developed in the gay community in North America would travel to Africa, and it did. In the 1980s, the majority of AIDS cases in South Africa were in white male homosexuals[2], so South Africa was a reasonable place for the Western gay discourse to enter Africa. However, it did not really take root there until the late 1990s with the birth of the Treatment Action Campaign, begun in 1998 by Zackie Achmat, a gay South African man with AIDS. By then the majority of AIDS cases in South Africa were in heterosexual blacks.

The question – apparently not asked at the time – was whether the mostly gay white American discourse of AIDS would be effective in the mostly heterosexual black African epidemic.

There are reasons to believe the gay discourse would apply. Homosexuals had been marginalized by the mainstream American community; Africans had been marginalized by the world community. Each of these "other" communities had a right to be heard on its own terms by the mainstream communities, and it appeared that a postmodern sensibility allowed for this. But there was yet another reason to expect the gay discourse to resonate in Africa, also stemming from a postmodern analysis. Questions of power and knowledge (mentioned in the Prologue) lie at the core of postmodernism: who has the power to determine what will be accepted as valid knowledge. Gays have for a long time been questioning the "knowledge" that said they were abnormal or perverted; Africans have likewise been suspicious of the "knowledge" that said they were primitive or wild. Yet in the "modern" world, neither group had the power to establish their self-understanding as standard "knowledge". Once again, it was postmodern thinking that questioned who defined what "knowledge" was, that exposed the power relations behind knowledge creation, and that proposed that there were other "knowledges."

These are the reasons why the North American gay discourse *should* apply to African AIDS. It is perhaps too early to decide how well it actually does fit, but we should at least engage the question. Prior to this we need to ask whether or not the gay discourse on AIDS was really a "foreign import". "There is a sense," says Megan Vaughan in *Curing Their Ills: Colonial Power and African Illness*, "in which colonial people and marginal groups in metropolitan societies discovered the postmodernist subject long before a postmodernist theory of subjectivity was elaborated in academic and literary circles. The experience of being a fragmented and fluid self was, if Fanon is correct, a common experience of colonial people as it was, according to many feminist writers, a common experience for women in Western societies."[3] And, we might add, gay people in the West. If this is true, the Western gay discourse should fit in Africa because it, or something like it, was already there.

However, it was not the postmodern discourse which first described AIDS in Africa, but the modern biomedical one – and this discourse was not flattering to Africa's "otherness". "In Europe and North America, both medical and journalistic accounts of AIDS in Africa indicated once again the durability of that European cultural tradition which sees Africa as synonymous with disease, death, and uncontrolled sexuality.... Africans have, of course, responded vigorously to this assault," sometimes seeing AIDS as predominantly a Western problem, and sometimes denying its existence altogether. But others "have steered away from this inversion. Rather than denying AIDS as a medical problem and projecting back on some 'Other', they emphasize rather the politico-economic context which has facilitated its spread in Africa." [4]

In other words, there is more than one "other" African voice; not surprisingly "otherness" is not monolithic. The question is how well these voices overlap with the gay activist discourse imported from the West. A corollary question is where Mbeki's voice fits among these other African voices. Let us begin with Mandisa Mbali, a South African AIDS activist with connections to the Treatment Action Coalition (TAC). Mbali's views are expressed in her 125-page history thesis, available on the internet. [5]

Mbali agrees with Vaughan that "AIDS discourse has been a repository of older ideas pathologising black and female sexuality, and 'homosexuality'." This approach, she suggests, was characteristic of the Apartheid era. However,

> in the post-apartheid era, there was a key shift towards rights-based discourse in family planning and AIDS policy-making, due to the work of key anti-apartheid left/liberal and feminist public health activists and academics, acting as historical agents. Despite this shift, Mbeki's denialism is a response to the largely extinct earlier colonial and late apartheid racist discourse around African sexuality as inherently diseased.

She describes this response further:

> In a broader philosophical sense though, recent post-apartheid fights over the science underpinning AIDS policy have been over who has scientific 'expertise', who has the right to speak authoritatively on science, what the scientific method is, and what constitutes valid scientific evidence. Instead of merely pointing to and condemning very real examples of racism in the history of AIDS, Mbeki appears to be attempting to throw out altogether the Western biomedical/scientific paradigm relating to AIDS as racist and neo-colonial. [6]

Mbeki may have a postmodern understanding of "otherness", she seems to be saying, but he has gone too far.

Mbali's judgment of Mbeki assumes he did deny the extent of AIDS in South Africa and the link between HIV and AIDS. Her analysis of Mbeki and her sources draw from the mainstream media presentation which, as we have seen, is controversial. As recently as May, 2003 (the controversy wouldn't die), another prominent South African weighed in. Writer and scholar Mbulelo Mzamane said,

> There was a yawning gulf, indeed, between what Mbeki actually said (www.gov.za) and how the media that was mischievous, at times, and downright incompetent, on occasion, reported the matter.... The rest of society largely took its cue from the media, which failed dismally to educate and inform the public on the issues.... We cannot agree that the South African government sowed nothing but confusion on the issue – the media did.[7]

Nevertheless, Mbali's analysis points to something very important. As we have seen in Chapters Three and Four, there are other critiques of the biomedical/scientific paradigm which do not necessarily result in denialism. Oyunga Pala's poignant question in

Chapter One, "Are we satisfied – or to what extent are we satisfied – with the answers which the scientific establishment has offered regarding HIV/AIDS medical theory and development?" is a fine example. It should also be clear by now that treatment activists must be deeply rooted in the biomedical/scientific paradigm, their major question being not "How do we treat AIDS?" but "Are these treatments readily available?" The gay activist discourse, in affirming its own "otherness", stops short of questioning the biomedical paradigm – and here African treatment activists seem to follow suite. Yet as we have seen, there are good reasons to critique the biomedical paradigm.

However, we must here consider a note of caution concerning postmodern analysis from an African philosopher, especially as we consider how well the Western gay activist discourse fits in Africa. Emmanuel Katongole, whose contributions at the Nkozi conference we reviewed in the last chapter, developed some of those ideas more fully in an academic article for *Modern Theology*. Here he uncovered an uncomfortable side effect of the postmodern celebration of difference. In a time of plentiful travel and communication, with

> different cultures and cultural artifacts that the post-liberal media puts before us for our 'info-tainment', differences are easily stripped of their moral and historical claims, and become merely 'aesthetic' – another aspect (commodity) for the post-liberal individual to enjoy, especially if he lives in the rich countries of the North.... As a result, what is promoted is a very superficial celebration of particularity, what one might call a frivolous fascination with difference."

Hence, he suggests, "there is something sinister about the postmodern celebration of difference, which at the same time renders difference ineffectual or inconsequential." In fact, he even suggests that "postmodernism involves a determination to destroy whatever is particular and local."[8]

If every option is possible, then every option is at the same time trivialized. The philosophical "permission" for gays to proclaim their difference – and for Africans to proclaim theirs – may be hollow. "A postmodern interest in African culture may not be liberating," he says. "What is needed, instead, is a more deeply entrenched theological practice which can challenge the different histories and politics which tend to obscure the actual historical struggles, conflicts and aspirations of the African peoples." The next section looks at some of these African theological foundations.

Theology

For us to understand African thought patterns better, it is necessary first to summarize some Western assumptions.

An overarching fact of the West, and especially North America, is our diversity. Our philosophical foundations may be in Greece and our theological foundations in Rome, but North American people come from all over the world. We may all agree on the techniques of microbiology and pharmacology, but we do not all use their products: witness the huge "alternative" health industry in the US. Most of us may be cultural descendants of the mediaeval European church, but many of us are not Christians. In order to live together we need some common ground.

Politically, democracy provides us with a system that imposes nothing on us except the will of the majority; religiously we have separated church from state; culturally the media bind us together, at least superficially. But we are still fundamentally diverse, and need a principle to allow that. Philosophically—articulated most clearly in medical ethics—we have that principle: autonomy. "I think, therefore I am" is our mantra, usually unspoken. Each of us, we believe, is a free moral agent, responsible ultimately only to him- or her-self. When confronted with someone who is fundamentally different from me, I can make no assumptions about how that other person should act, other than obeying the laws. Precisely because we have no philosophical beliefs in common, individual autonomy becomes our common ground.

This radical autonomy has different effects on different people. Some reject the diversity, and call those different from them "wrong". Some celebrate the diversity and the options it presents. But underneath, many of us find a very fine line between being autonomously alone and being lonely. In that loneliness we sometimes become preoccupied with meaning—or its lack—and with the end of everything, death. Stronger than our desire to live life is our desire to avoid death and—especially in medicine—we do all we can to avoid it. Our fear becomes our focus.

It is these two principles—**autonomy** and preoccupation with **death**—which gives us some perspective in understanding two pivotal aspects of African philosophy: **community** and **life**.

> African ethics is not concerned about respect for one's own self: the community occupies center stage in such a way that the individual members must always bear in mind and aim at growth in quality and life for all members... [N]o one can realize himself as a person all by himself; one becomes a person only in relationship to others.[9]

> The foundation and purpose of the ethical perspective of African Religion is life, life in its fullness. Everything is perceived with reference to this.... Does the particular happening promote life? If so, it is good, just, ethical, desirable, divine. Or, does it diminish life in any way? Then it is wrong, bad, unethical, unjust, detestable.[10]

These two concepts of **life** in **community** come together in the ubuntu ("humanity") theology popularized by Desmond Tutu.[11]

Most important for our discussion is the understanding that life in community continues after physical death. "While the departed person is remembered by name, he is not really dead: he is alive, and such a person I would call the *living-dead*. The living-dead is a person who is physically dead but alive in the memory of those who knew him in his life as well as being alive in the world of the spirits."[12]

116

We can see the importance of understanding these philosophical concepts when we look at the difference between the Western attitudes that see ARVs as pivotal in the fight against AIDS, and the African attitudes which are cooler toward them. For Westerners preoccupied with avoiding death, ARVs are critical because they do exactly that—they postpone death. Further, even though not every HIV+ person can or should use them, each autonomous person needs to be given that choice. For many Africans, however, life is much larger than biological life, and includes the life of the community and life with the ancestors. The physical death of the individual does not need to be avoided at all cost, especially when that avoidance is simply a postponement of physical death, and the cost imperils others. The quote above refers to promoting life and diminishing life, not prolonging life or avoiding death. Some African people that I have discussed this with are far more concerned with the life of the community—i.e., preventive activities—than the postponement of the death of an individual with drugs. Although this perspective may be weakening as more Africans move to cities and the influence of traditional values wanes, there is still a remarkable resilience of African traditional values.

Keeping these general principles in mind, we will now turn to some specific theological reflections on AIDS by two of the authors just quoted. They both predate the Mbeki controversy by nearly a decade, and give us some foundation to see that controversy more clearly.

In 1992, Laurenti Magesa, the writer quoted above who referred to "life in its fullness", published "AIDS and Survival in Africa: A Tentative Reflection".[13] This was the last chapter in a collection of essays by African authors entitled *Moral and Ethical Issues in African Christianity*—published, by the way, only in Africa. Magesa is a Catholic priest and moral theologian, sometimes serving as a parish priest in Tanzanian villages, sometimes teaching in African or US universities.

He begins with an observation which is still true 12 years later: "Two distinct tendencies characterize discourse on Aids in Africa. One tendency caricatures the continent and all but defines Africa in terms of the epidemic.... The other is a more respectful and respectable approach..., [recognizing] Aids is a problem 'with social and political causes and hence in theory resoluble.'" The difference between caricature and a respectful approach, between appearance and reality, understandably belongs at the beginning of a theological reflection.

He then suggests three ways to understand AIDS in Africa, three "cosmologies". The first is the traditional one, where people see AIDS as a matter of magic and taboo, with the appropriate response being ritual. While this view still clearly influences how people behave, it is "inadequate from the contemporary standpoint... there can be no going back completely to that cosmological view." Second, there is the modern view, which sees AIDS linked to sexual activity, with the appropriate response sexual continence. While this is clearly a reasonable goal, in 1992 Magesa doubted that it was the predominant cosmology of most Africans. The number of AIDS cases was—and still is—rising across the continent; for many Africans the direct link between AIDS and sexual activity, *and the response to limit sexual activity,* had clearly not yet happened.

In between these two cosmologies Magesa proposed a third approach, which did see AIDS as "directly linked to sexual activity," but with people responding in a "confused" or "muddled" way. "In response to the threat of certain death caused by the disease, [their] behavior is not appropriate; it indicates nonchalance or even helplessness." It is this cosmology, "the confused view," which Magesa sees as predominating in Africa today. He then goes on to consider which countries are most affected by AIDS, seeming to leave behind the question of cosmology. However, his discussion of "the Aids map of Africa" leads back directly to why people might be confused.

Magesa notes that while "massive socio-political upheavals" and poverty both are important in the spread of AIDS, these factors alone cannot account for why some regions are heavily affected, and other much less so. He then proposes that religion is an important factor: places with low AIDS prevalence "have either a predominantly Muslim or a non-Western (deeply indigenous)

Christian influence." In contrast, places with high AIDS prevalence "have a predominantly Western Christian influence." The point, however, is not that the doctrines or practices of Islam are more AIDS-protective than those of Christianity; they are in fact similar. Rather, Islam "adapted itself more readily and much more thoroughly to significant aspects of African traditional view of sex and sexuality." Christianity, on the other hand, "was overwhelmed by its Western cultural medium, and negated and undermined in real life what it taught in theory. Thus, while not consciously intending it, Western Christianity seems to have encouraged in Africa an unprecedented libertarian sexual behavior. Contrary to the African communitarian, taboo and ritual cosmological approaches, sexual relations came to be seen as a private matter of the individuals concerned. The consequences of the use of one's sexual powers to the community of the living and the dead faded into the background." This unhealthy mixture of Christianity and Western culture led in Africa to the "confused" cosmology he previously mentioned.

Clearly, since the problem of AIDS is multi-factorial, the solutions need to be as well. Magesa suggests the "central concern in the campaign to contain the epidemic" is behavior modification, approached in two ways: structural changes (economic development, political stability, control of sex-tourism, and improved health systems) and a moral or ethical approach. However, this ethical approach must be rooted in "traditional African cosmology"—not "to resurrect a dead past" but "to seriously take cultural elements still extant in the African social psyche" because "completely alien, borrowed solutions will hardly work." He then summarizes what must be at the core of an African-rooted approach: "Besides the profound sense of God and the hereafter, [there is] the perception of life as the ultimate good and... community as the context of the possibility of human existence." This one sentence condenses the essence of African philosophy and provides a framework to judge any approach to control AIDS in Africa.

The other African theologian quoted above, the one who said "community occupies center stage" in African ethics, is Benezet

Bujo, a Congolese Catholic priest who has taught in African universities, and is now teaching in Switzerland. In 1993 he published some ethical reflections on community in German, which came out in English 1998 as *The Ethical Dimension of Community: The African Model and the Dialogue Between North and South.* Near the end of this book was his chapter on AIDS: "The Importance of the Community for Ethical Action: the Example of AIDS".[14]

For Bujo, as noted above, community is foundational in an understanding of African cosmology. "The individual knows himself or herself to be immersed in the community to such an extent that personality can develop only in and through it." Consequently, "because no clan member can live in unrelatedness, in cases of misfortune the cause is looked for within the community itself. According to African wisdom, a disease is always an indication that something in human relations is wrong." Later in the chapter, Bujo makes it clear that since AIDS is an international disease, it is reasonable to apply these principles internationally: "the problem of this disease is not an individual question alone, but possibly first of all a structural one." The community here is the entire world, and the disordered structures Bujo sees are the ones we have previously discussed: unjust economic policies "established by the Northern countries", poverty, Third World debt, etc.

Naturally, "the reformation of our society is a task which cannot be mastered by the individual alone." Yet "in the discussion concerning AIDS, one often gets the impression that prevention of this epidemic is possible if the individual behaves more carefully." Then using his own thoughts together with quotes from others, Bujo shows the inadequacy of an individual behavior-change approach:

> 'If an information campaign is satisfied with advertising condoms, without exposing the deeper causes and ignoring the ethical questions, then one is merely treating the symptoms.' Advertising condoms rather promotes the consumer mentality, reducing sexuality to a commodity.... Only an ethical conviction is able to fight this consumer

mentality efficiently and to restore sexuality its dignity....
'Neither purely technical advice (use condoms, prevent
AIDS!) nor moral admonitions (remain faithful!) are
sufficient to control the disease. The prevention and
stopping of AIDS does not depend solely on the individual
but on the quality of our institutions, changes in culture,
economy and politics as well.'

Note carefully: Bujo is not against condoms because the church
requires him to be. In fact, neither he nor Magesa rules out the use
of condoms. He is rather cautioning against individual approaches
to a disease which has communal causes. He is, like Katongole in
the previous chapter, concerned with "condomization" and its
effects on Africa. Bujo puts it this way: "From an African
perspective, it is to be stated that an indiscriminate distribution of
condoms ultimately wipes out African culture." He is arguing here
as an African, not a priest. In fact, mentioning aspects of African
tradition which "prepare for sexual self-discipline", he writes that
"colonial policy *and European Christianity* have already destroyed
this cultural background a lot.... If the industrialized nations wish
to help Africa, they should offer their support in such a way that
the African people can recover their spiritual and moral immunity,
which cannot be underestimated even if it does not offer or replace
a technical solution for AIDS." (My emphasis.)

Ultimately, this loss of one of the vital elements of traditional
African culture hurts not only Africa, but the entire world
community. "The African community understands itself as a
healing community", but this self understanding is under threat.
When Western medicine was brought to Africa by the colonists, it

> ...was never integrated into people's consciousness;
> [rather] colonial systems destroyed the African medical
> tradition, which could no longer be effectively applied. For
> even if the Western type of medicine proved to be more
> efficient in many cases, the holistic approach to medicine
> was lost, since the modern method of treatment looked at

the person merely from the viewpoint of 'repairing' one's organs.

Bujo is clearly not a "dissident": he believes there is an AIDS virus, and admits there are "efficient" Western technical solutions. His critique, like that of Owa-Mataze and Kanyandago and Katongole and Magesa, is rooted in his understanding of Africa, and thus is far deeper than the Western dissident critique. The question for these scholars is not merely the nature of the microbe or where it came from or whether the statistics are precisely accurate, but rather the overall cultural approach to health and disease. Their questions are not aimed at the findings of science, but how we use it. Their concern is not whether or not an individual uses a condom, but rather what is ignored when condoms become the essence of prevention.

Gender

In 1998 I met a young American woman in Nairobi who had been doing some short term volunteer work in Western Kenya with AIDS education. She told me her feminist perspective: that AIDS was a gender issue, and that African women were the victims in this epidemic. I listened politely, and then told her (relying on my decade of clinical experience in Africa) that AIDS was simply a sexually transmitted disease—that men infected women, and that women infected men. I communicated gently enough that she listened, but internally I was annoyed that yet again a Western ideology was being superimposed on African experience. I had not heard this gender analysis from Africans, and simply assumed it was a Western misreading of an African problem.

Five years later, in preparation for a trip to Africa related to this book, I read as much as I could find from African authors about their understanding of AIDS—and once again, found little from a gender perspective. There were of course the Western feminist readings similar to what I had heard in 1998, but almost nothing that I could find written by Africans. However, when I arrived back in Africa, the conversations I had with African scholars and AIDS workers in late 2003 contained a surprise for me. Men were talking about the gender issue and were telling me it was important. Several conversations—including some with women theologians—underlined for me the vitality of the gender discourse in Africa. And when I read African novels that touch on AIDS, it became very clear that gender is one of the key elements in the African understandings of AIDS.

The essence of this discourse, as we shall see, confirmed what the young American woman had told me in 1998—that women are to some extent the victims in African AIDS. But it wasn't the content of the discourse that was a surprise. The involvement of men, the contribution of theologians, the perspective of novelists, together with my difficulty finding things written by Africans on a feminist interpretation of AIDS, all suggest to me that in Africa, gender is not a "women's issue"; it's an issue about power and about sexuality; it's a human issue. Admittedly there is much overlap between the African gender discourse and a Western feminist perspective. But, as with the Western dissident discourse, the overlap is not complete. The following, drawn solely from African sources, are some ways to view gender issues in African AIDS.

One assumption in gender discussions is that the fundamental issue is power: "Progress can only be brought about by addressing power imbalance between genders in all spheres of life."[15] But what is the origin of this power imbalance in Africa? One approach suggests that a fundamental problem is African culture itself. Anna Mary Mukamwezi Kayonga says, "In most African cultures women are mere slaves who are there to look after children and be treated like dirt.... On the whole the majority of African women are oppressed." She then gives some examples from the traditional practices in several African ethnic groups, and concludes, "All in all, the whole socio-cultural framework in Africa is male. The existing structures are used as vehicles for the submission of women, who are trodden underfoot by men at every level."[16] The overlap here with Western feminism is evident, and there is undoubtedly much true in this analysis.

However, there is another view of traditional African culture. While agreeing that there is currently a power imbalance between genders, Kariuki Thuku of the Kenyan Community Peace Museums Programme suggests this was not always so. Using examples from traditional sexual education in Agikuyu culture, he shows that "sexuality is not an independent statute in the African traditions", but rather "is intricately embedded in our cultural veins and arteries and it does obey the law of collective responsibility." In other words, sexuality did not always exist in the context of imbalance of power. "Girls and boys were equipped with the power of language and visual art necessary when confronting discussions and debates on sexuality."

Unfortunately, the traditional language and symbols of sexuality are being lost, and

> ...lack of a morally and socially accepted sexuality language is a big drawback in the fight against HIV/AIDS.... The fear arising from the lack of sexually accepted terminologies has [made women] weak, defenseless and unmentionably incapable of brilliantly confronting and winning a sexually related argument. This phenomenon has robbed our women of their 'power, pride, and dignity of fertility'; it has purged them into a state of sexual servitude... our women are financially disenfranchised, ... sexuality... is being held ransom by men.[17]

The Minister of Health in South Africa comes to a similar conclusion by a different route. "[T]hose traditional institutions," she says, "...that provided the 'holy basis' for the principles of manhood, like circumcision schools, have themselves been invaded by forces of darkness and now cannot be trusted to deliver... even though they used to be the guardians of culture values and norms in the olden days."[18]

The debate here is not whether or not there is a current power imbalance. The question is the role of culture: did the imbalance come about *because* of African culture, or because of the *loss* of some of its key elements? Though there is clearly evidence for both, we must be very cautious of the matter of *blame* in choosing one or the other, as we saw with articles in the *New African*. Emphasizing the role of African culture in gender power imbalance seems to put the blame on Africa; emphasizing the loss of some of the key elements in traditional African culture as the cause puts the blame more on those forces, often Western, which have helped to destroy African culture.

Regardless of how the power imbalance came about, it is there— and can lead to women being victims in the AIDS epidemic. Constance Shisanya, who lectures at Kenyatta University, describes it this way:

> Most communities in Kenya prohibit married women from having lovers. Men, on the other hand, are free to engage in extra marital sexual relationships since polygyny is condoned.... To this end, many women are victims of their husbands' irresponsible sexual behaviors... in most cases, men infect their wives [with HIV] since culturally the latter have little or no control over their sexuality. This is because the payment of bride wealth, in most communities in Kenya, places women in defenseless situations whereby they are expected to meet their husbands' sexual demands all the time.... The pervasive threat of physical violence or divorce makes women to surrender to unsafe sex with their husbands. Unfortunately, those women who suspect that their spouses could be HIV seropositive have got no way of protecting themselves from the epidemic through the use of condoms since men in Kenya are the ones who decide whether or not a contraceptive should be used.

And finally,

> Economic factors equally make women in Kenya more vulnerable to HIV/AIDS than men.... The inability of some women to provide basic necessities to their children has led them to engage in risky activities such as prostitution

125

with a view to surviving now rather than leaving their children to die of hunger. Yet multiple sexual partners expose an individual to the possibility of HIV/AIDS infection.[19]

Botswanan theologian Musa Dube summarizes the same material this way:

A major factor in the spread of HIV/Aids is the powerlessness of women: their incapacity to make decisions about their lives due to the lack of material ownership and decision making powers.... [We cannot] turn a blind eye to the structures that make abstaining, being faithful, and condomizing, *not* as easy as ABC! When our relationships are based on gender, race and class inequalities, fighting HIV/Aids is more than just abstaining, being faithful and condomizing.[20]

This gender analysis, as Dube has just pointed out, leads to the uncomfortable conclusion that the standard AIDS control measures simply don't work. Shisanya agrees: "The awareness campaigns... have not yielded fruits since the spread of HIV/AIDS continues unabated." A Tanzanian scholar, Beth Maina Ahlberg, feels the same way: "There is increasing evidence that AIDS educational campaigns have generally resulted in increased information but little change in behavior."[21] Preventing AIDS is *not* as easy as ABC. One obvious response, of course, is to broaden the prevention campaign. Shisanya suggests that "addressing the imbalances in power between men and women in Kenyan communities" is a critical step in controlling AIDS. This involves religious and cultural and economic and legal changes—much larger tasks than simply ABC, but tasks that are necessary when ABC alone is not working.

However, as we noted above, gender issues are not *only* about power. Ahlberg's analysis takes us in a somewhat different, though not contradictory, direction. Instead of focusing on gender power imbalances, she looks at the "moral regimes" which influence the sexual behavior of both men and women. She refers to the same moral confusion as Magesa, outlining four moral regimes in contemporary Africa: the Christian, the traditional African, the administrative/legal, and the secular 'romantic love'. Many of the AIDS education programs are based on the first three, all of which discourage pre-marital sexual activity. But many young people "embrace the 'romantic love' moral regime which dictates that sexual activity is all right so long as people are in love, regardless of their marital status." This often involves serial monogamy, and within each relationship "adolescents may not practice safe sex, simply because they consider themselves at no risk: their relationship at that particular time is firm and involves just one faithful partner." There is consequently a disjuncture between the moral regimes behind the adult world designing the AIDS programs, and the moral regime of many of the people at risk of AIDS—leading, of course, to the confusion that Magesa mentioned.

I saw this confusion in an edition of the Uganda *Monitor*, October 3, 2003. On the front page was an article titled "First Lady cautions on use of condoms" in which Mrs. Museveni is quoted as saying, "I am not comfortable with the thought that the [fate] of an entire continent could depend upon a thin piece of rubber". On the second page the headline article was "Law on malicious Aids infection due," reporting on legislation regarding people who knowingly infect others with AIDS. These articles clearly reflect the African and administrative/legal moral regimes just noted. However, the magazine section in the center of the same edition contained in its "Sex Talk" column an article titled "No Hard Rules Here," written by a woman, which talked about techniques of sex, not its context. The entire weekly pull-out section (titled *Women & Men*) was full of articles, written by both women and men, rooted in the secular 'romantic love' moral regime. And in the "Lonely Hearts" column, two of the eleven personals said the person they were looking for should be willing to undergo an HIV test—acknowledging, but not closing, the gap between moral regimes.

Yet simply preaching "safe sex" in this context has not worked. "It is clear," says Ahlberg, "that, if there is to be any success in the control of HIV/AIDS..., there is a dire need to address the paradoxical situation of silence and prohibition.... What is required is an approach which makes people recognize themselves" —i.e., one rooted in their 'idealized past'.

> In this case, it would be more appropriate to tell the Kikuyu people that they once had an open sexual model which protected adolescents engaging in sexual activity outside of marriage, rather than telling them to change from their inherently permissive and unchanged sexuality. In this context, we are calling for an education system which focuses on people's history.[22]

Here, Ahlberg sidesteps the question of whether African culture or its loss is the cause of present gender imbalances; she simply asserts that to be effective, educational programs must be rooted in what people know. Local history, she says, "is an important entry point in generating open dialogue, as it activates people's meanings rather than attempting to confirm assumptions which have racial and cultural prejudices."

As mentioned earlier, I had some difficulty finding articles written from an African gender perspective. However, a draft of an article by Nobantu Rasebotsa on "AIDS Fiction in Africa"[23] pointed me to the works of African novelists. Prof. Rasebotsa, who admits that she writes from a feminist perspective, is a professor of English at the University of Botswana. When I read some of the novels she had analyzed, together with several others, I found a surprise: virtually every novel I read concerning AIDS, some written by men and others by women, had a female main character—sometimes a "victim", yet at the same time usually a strong woman, committed to doing what she could to slow the spread of AIDS. The last chapter will look closely at some of these novels.

REFERENCES

[1] **Sabatier, Renee (1988),** *Blaming Others: Prejudice, Race and Worldwide AIDS* (Washington, DC, Panos and New Society Publishers); **Farmer,**

Paul (1992), *AIDS and Accusation: Haiti and the Geography of Blame* (Berkeley, University of California Press).

[2]**Maartens, G, Wood, R, O'Keefe, E, and Byrne, C (1997)**, "Independent epidemics of heterosexual and homosexual HIV infection in South Africa—survival differences", *Q J Med* 1997; 90:449-454.

[3] **Vaughan, Megan (1991)**, *Curing Their Ills: Colonial Power and African Illness* (Stanford, Stanford University Press) p. 204.

[4] **Vaughan**, *Ibid.*, p. 205-6, **(1991)**.

[5] **Mbali, Mandisa (2001)**, *"A Long Illness": Towards a History of NGO, Government and Medical discourse around AIDS policy-making in South Africa, www.history.und.ac.za/grad.asp*

[6] **Mbali**, *Ibid.*, Abstract, p. 72, **(2001)**.

[7] **Mzamane, Mbulelo (2003)**, "HIV/Aids and the politics of the new South Africa,"
http://www.africanreviewofbooks.com/Newsitems/mzamane.html

[8] **Katongole, Emmanuel (2000b)**, "Postmodern Illusions and the Challenges of African Theology: The Ecclesial Tactics of Resistance," *Modern Theology* 16:2 April, p.237-254.

[9] **Bujo, Benezet (2001)**, *Foundations of an African Ethic: Beyond the Universal Claims of Western Morality*, (New York, Crossroad Publishing Co), p. 60, 88.

[10] **Magesa, Laurenti (1997)**, *African Religion: The Moral Traditions of Abundant Life*, (Maryknoll, N.Y., Orbis Books), p. 77.

[11] See, for example, **Michael Battle's (1977)** *Reconciliation: The Ubuntu Theology of Desmond Tutu*, (Cleveland, Ohio, Pilgrim Press).

[12] **Mbiti, John (1969)**, *African Religions and Philosophy*, (Nairobi, East African Educational Publishers), p. 25.

[13] **Magesa, Laurenti (1992)**, "Aids and Survival in Africa: A Tentative

Reflection," in *Moral and Ethical Issues in African Christianity: A Challenge for African Christianity,* ed by J.N.K. Mugambi and A. Nasimiyu-Wasike (Nairobi, Acton Publishers, reprinted 2003.), p. 197-216.

[14] **Bujo, Benezet (1998),** *The Ethical Dimension of Community: The African Model and the Dialogue Between North and South* (Nairobi, Paulines Publications Africa), p. 181-195.

[15] **Shisanya, Constance (2001),** "The Impact of HIV/AIDS on Women in Kenya," *Quests for Abundant Life in Africa,* ed. by Mary N Getui and Matthew M Theuri (Acton Publishers, Nairobi) p. 45-64.

[16] **Kayonga, Anna Mary Mukamwezi (1992),** "African Women and Morality," in *Moral and Ethical Issues in African Christianity: A Challenge for African Christianity,* ed by J.N.K. Mugambi and A. Nasimiyu-Wasike (Acton Publishers, Nairobi, reprinted 2003.), p. 140-143.

[17] **Thuku, Kariuki (2003),** "Peace is Health: Agikuyu Forest Symbols of Sexuality," *unpublished paper,* 2003.

[18] **Tshabalala-Msimang, Manto (2002),** "Opening Address≅ in *ASouth Africa Men Care Enough to Act":* Report, *National Men=s Imbizo on HIV/AIDS, 4-5 October, 2002,* published by Department of Health, South Africa., p. 14-16.

[19] **Shisanya,** *op. cit.* p. 50-53, **(2001).**

[20] **Dube, Musa (2001),** "Unsettling the Christian Church," *Reformed World,* vol 51, no. 4, December.

[21] **Ahlberg, Beth Maina (1994),** "Is There a Distinct African Sexuality? A Critical response to Caldwell," *Africa* 64 (2), p. 221-235.

[22] **Ahlberg,** *Ibid.,* **1994.**

[23] **Rasebotsa, Nobantu (2004),** "AIDS Fiction in Africa" in *The Discourse of Hiv/Aids in Africa,* edited by Emevwo Biakolo, Joyce Mathangwane, and Dan Odallo, (Pretoria and Gabarone, UNAIDS.)

6

The African Press:
Reporting the African AIDS Discourse

Before looking at African fiction writers, however, we will take a brief look specifically at African journalists. Although I have quoted from the African press repeatedly throughout this book, I would like to use a single recent event and its context as a case study of how the African media saw this event, and how their reporting suggests some distinctly African understandings.

First, the context. On May 27, 2003, when US President George W. Bush signed a $15 billion package to fight AIDS in Africa, he said:

> We know how to prevent AIDS, and we know how to treat it. The cost of effective medicines has fallen dramatically. And we made progress here in our own country.... We will also help the people across Africa who are struggling against this disease....[1]

Just over a month later, on July 2, 2003, he appointed Randy Tobias, former CEO of the Eli Lilly pharmaceutical company, as his "Global AIDS Coordinator". During the appointment ceremony Bush summarized the US approach to AIDS:

> We'll work quickly to get help to the people who need it most by purchasing low-cost, anti-retroviral medications and other drugs that are needed to save lives. We will set up a broad and efficient network to deliver drugs to the farthest reaches of Africa, even by motorcycle or bicycle.
>
> We will train doctors and nurses and other health care professionals so they can treat HIV/AIDS patients. Our efforts will ensure that clinics and laboratories will be built or renovated and then equipped. Child care workers will

131

be hired and trained to care for AIDS orphans, and people living with AIDS will get home-based care to ease their suffering.

Throughout all regions of the targeted countries we will provide HIV testing. We will support abstinence-based prevention education. Faith-based and community organizations will have our help as they provide treatment and prevention and support services in communities affected by HIV/AIDS. And we're developing a system to monitor and evaluate this entire program, so we can be sure we're getting the job done.[2]

Few people would consider George Bush an expert on African AIDS—though his AIDS package did win rapid bipartisan support in the United States congress. AIDS workers were generally surprised, and pleased, at the substantial amount of money the Bush administration was offering to spend on African AIDS. Some were admittedly worried that his emphasis on "abstinence-based" programs would inhibit their "condom-based" prevention programs. Others were upset that he did not offer the bulk of the package to the already existing UN Global AIDS Fund. Nevertheless, the essence of his program—prevention education, biomedical treatment, and care for orphans and those living with AIDS—reflects the standard Western approach to AIDS. To reinforce this approach, Bush traveled through several African countries for a week in July, 2003.

The event we will look at, which followed Bush's visit to Africa, was an international AIDS conference, one of over half a dozen listed by UNAIDS. These are big conferences, with thousands of attendees, many of them scientists, sharing their latest discoveries. They have the support of major international scientific organizations, and funding from huge multinational pharmaceutical companies. Many specific conferences are held every year or two; since 2001 we have already had the Fourth International Conference on HIV/AIDS in Women and Children, the Sixth European Conference of Experimental AIDS Research, the Eleventh International Conference for People Living with AIDS, the

Twelfth International Symposium on HIV and Emerging Infections, and the Fourteenth International AIDS Conference. Central among these conferences, for this epidemic in which two-thirds of the disease burden is in Africa, was the Thirteenth ICASA — International Conference on AIDS and STDs in Africa, held in Nairobi September 21-26, 2003.

All of these conferences contain a great deal of information. The Nairobi ICASA, for example, had 6 conference "tracks", attempting to look at all aspects of AIDS: prevention, care, biomedical science, research and evaluation, national and community response, and finally cultural and ethical issues – the first four mirroring the elements noted above. Significantly at this conference, the majority of attendees were African. In other words, this conference would seem to be an excellent venue to find an African view of AIDS. It was: the majority of presenters were also African.

I arrived in Nairobi the day before the conference ended. I was at the beginning of a six week trip through east and southern Africa to talk with African scholars about how they understood AIDS. I did not attend the ICASA conference, and so cannot evaluate to what extent the content was distinctly African. I did see some television reports on the last two days of the conference, specifically about some HIV positive demonstrators outside the conference who were demanding anti-retroviral drugs. I was around for the next few weeks, however, and was able to see how the local media reported on this African conference.

What I read in the local papers confirmed my impression: what African reporters chose to write about often carried different emphases from what I read in the Western media. Of course they reported on the theme of the conference "Access to Care: Challenges", and carried several articles about various government plans to provide anti-retroviral drugs to people with AIDS. But sometimes they uncovered pieces of the story less likely to receive attention in the West; often they simply arranged their news reports in ways that made clear their concerns.

For example, the day after the conference opened, the Kenya *Nation* began an article on the conference this way:

As the ICASA conference got underway yesterday, it was clear that community groups have been embraced as key players at international conferences. Their non-scientific activities have been inserted into the conference programs as recognition that they are the 'engine' of future action in the battle against AIDS.[3]

To Bush, in the quote above, community organizations seem ancillary to the main thrust of getting drugs to people; to the *Nation*, community groups are the "engine" and the drugs, mentioned later in the article, are ancillary.

An equally interesting article, making a similar point, was in the Uganda *Monitor* the next day. Carolyne Nakazibwe, in an article about the conference, wrote, "Uganda's anti-AIDS campaign is still exemplary in Africa despite less than 10 percent of its patients having access to anti-retroviral therapy." She ended her article with a similar unique view of statistics: "Despite the pandemic's severity, UNAIDS notes that 90% of Africans do not have the virus that causes AIDS, raising the need to continue the preventive measures."[4]

Two days later the Africa Church Information Service released an article about traditional healers at ICASA. It read in part "African traditional healers have demanded recognition by governments and involvement in the management of HIV/AIDS pandemic in the continent," and then quoted a Senegalese traditional healer who noted that most sub-Saharan Africans used and believed in traditional medicine. "He [the traditional healer] called for a change in the mindset of people who considered traditional healing as inferior and primitive."[5] The mainstream Western approach, summarized above, mentions neither traditional healers, nor even cultural patterns and forces that may underlie the epidemic.

Several articles during and immediately after the conference pointed to the gender discussions that were taking place there. One pointed out that "male attitudes towards women and sex have long been acknowledged as one of the biggest sources of Africa's AIDS pandemic,"[6] another quoted Kenyan President Kibaki on the need "to empower women and ensure that their rights are protected,"[7] and a third was titled "Women Alone Can't Stop AIDS in Africa."[8]

This last article from *The East African Standard* contained the full text of a speech given by the UN Special Envoy for AIDS, Stephen Lewis. Why the *Standard* chose that particular speech to quote in full may be related to what Lewis said near the end:

> Africa needs no instructions from the West; Africa needs no arrogance from the West; Africa needs no churlish lectures from the West. Africans know HIV/AIDS in all its manifestations and requirements.... Africa has vastly more experience of orphans than the rest of us.... The knowledge and human resources are there: organizations of People Living With AIDS, the inspired youth peer counselors, the political leadership, the religious leadership, the activist women's groups, the community-based and faith-based organizations: there is overwhelming sophistication and strength on this continent.

This is a very different message than the West usually reports or hears; very different from Bush's "We will set up... we will train... our efforts will ensure... we're developing a system...." Lewis's conclusion: "What's missing are the tools and support to do the job...; that requires money." Period.

The next week the Uganda *Monitor* carried the previously-mentioned front-page article titled "First Lady Cautions on Use of Condoms," quoting Mrs. Janet Museveni: "I am not comfortable with the thought that the [fate] of an entire continent could depend upon a thin piece of rubber." The *Monitor* article was quoting from an opinion piece in a US newspaper by US Senator Lamar Alexander in which he had noted that Mrs. Museveni emphasized the value of A (abstinence) and B (being faithful) more than C (condoms) in the ABC approach. Alexander, in his comments on how to use the $15 billion from the US, "suggested using at least part of the money to dig wells... 'Since AIDS destroys immune systems, victims of all ages live longer with clean water,' he said."[9]

Once again, this broader understanding of the reasons behind the suffering of AIDS is notably absent from Bush's comments.

Finally, two weeks after the conference ended, *The East African*, a weekly newspaper covering Kenya, Uganda, and Tanzania, carried seven articles on AIDS. Only four referred directly to ICASA, but it was clear that the conference had made AIDS newsworthy again. The first article, on page 4, dealt with the research of American Prof David Gisselquist (a speaker at ICASA), who's findings suggested that as much as 30% of African AIDS was due to needle contamination. The article then quoted WHO official Dr. Paulo Teixeira as saying that only 5-7% of AIDS was from unsafe medical practices. However, earlier WHO reports had put the figure at 2.4%. *The East African's* conclusion was that Gisselquist's research "has provoked the World Health Organization into updating its rates of infection through needles and other unsafe medical practices from 2.4 to 7 per cent even while denouncing the research findings."[10]

On page 6 were two more articles, one on Kenya buying anti-retroviral drugs[11], and the other on a laboratory supplier complaining that his company was overlooked by the Kenyan Ministry of Health.[12] In the sports section was an article reporting on sports stars who were vocal in their attempts to publicize the fight against AIDS, and suggesting they could do more.[13] And in the Magazine Section of the paper was a report on a presentation by children at ICASA on their struggles and understandings of AIDS. The article acknowledged that Kenyan President Kibaki "last week launched an ambitious program to halve the price of anti-retroviral (ARV) drugs in Kenya," but continued:

> Yet while much of the attention at ICASA was focused on ARVs, more grassroots issues were being addressed at dozens of small 'satellite sessions'.... On the first day of the conference, a groundbreaking study on Africa's youth was launched by a group of confident young children from the slums of Kibera."

The rest of the article was on the risks children face, but also on the hope that they (not ARVs) bring.[14]

Finally there were two opinion columns about AIDS. The first did not refer specifically to ICASA, but rather to Kenyan President Kibaki's upcoming visit to the US, suggesting what Kibaki should tell Bush about AIDS. Regarding treatment, the author saw no reason for Bush to set up "a new American HIV/AIDS global disbursement mechanism that will in effect compete with the [UN] Global Fund," especially as the American fund would be "headed by Randal Tobias of Eli Lilly and Co, one of the multinational pharmaceutical companies that lead the lobby in favor of patent protection under the WTO." Then "with respect to prevention, the Bush administration has pursued an abstinence-only approach that pays no attention to African women's inability to insist on an abstinence-only approach. In fact, by denying funding to African organizations that focus on African women's reproductive and sexual rights, the Bush administration has placed African women under threat." [15]

The second column dealt with the demonstrators outside the ICASA conference, the ones demanding anti-retroviral treatment. While conferences are sometimes marginally newsworthy, demonstrators are usually given headlines. Certainly previous South African demonstrators advocating for treatment have been well covered by the Western press, and their leader, Zackie Achmat, has even been nominated for the Nobel Peace Prize[16]. How did the African press see the Nairobi demonstrators? They were certainly covered, both in the print media and on the local television. Articles and interviews with the activists explored their concerns, namely that at present antiretrovirals were difficult to obtain in most African settings, and that they should be provided for those with AIDS.

The opinion column in *The East African* reviewed these concerns, and essentially agreed with them. However, the title of the article conveyed the author's perspective: "Activists of the World, Chill Out, and We've Heard You." He suggested that while some African governments have in the past ignored AIDS,

...it is also true that many governments on the continent have woken up to the ravages of the disease, mounting commendable efforts with extremely limited resources to contain the disease.... Listening to activists from the so-called international NGOs talk, one wouldn't know this. Their take is invariably on how corrupt Aids control councils are, or how inept African governments have been in responding to the crisis.

The author likewise defended the pharmaceutical companies for what progress they had made so far, while still agreeing they should not "be let off the hook."

As for career HIV/Aids activists, they urgently need to shift focus from bashing the drug firms and shouting themselves hoarse over patents to more constructive engagements. Top among these is to lobby corporate bodies in hard-hit countries to start workplace treatment programs....[17]

The activists deserved to be heard, and deserved a rebuttal, which was printed in the following week's *East African*, written by a Kenyan. It defended the need to keep pressure on the pharmaceutical companies.[18] However, it is not simply the facts of what the companies were or were not doing that bothered the author of the "Chill Out" article. He felt that the approach of the activists was foreign; he said "many of them [were] 30-somethings from rich Nordic countries." The day after I arrived in Nairobi I asked a Kenyan professor what he thought of the activists. He said, "They came from somewhere. Someone brought them in." Three weeks later I met an official of the ICASA conference during a discussion with another Kenyan scholar. I asked the official about the activists. "Oh," she said, "the ones who came up from South Africa? They asked our permission to demonstrate, and we agreed. We were glad the police didn't stop them." The activists were indeed African, but what bothered the *East African* writer was that their style was not.

It is interesting that an American group would nominate an African activist for the Nobel Peace Prize, while an African commentator would tell similar activists in his country to "chill out". It takes an African journalist to point out that African women are unable to insist on an "abstinence only" approach to AIDS prevention. It is noteworthy that a Ugandan journalist would celebrate her country's AIDS program despite only 10% of AIDS patients being on ARVs. It is fascinating that an African journalist would report on a disputed study on rates of HIV infection from contaminated needles, and then conclude that WHO had "updated" its rates. It is significant that the opinions of a US Senator from a minor US newspaper appear as front page news in Uganda. In fact, Western and African commentators see the same disease quite differently. There is a distinctly "African discourse", as these press reports show.

References

[1] *http://www.whitehouse.gov/news/releases/2003/05/20030527-7.html*

[2] *http://www.whitehouse.gov/news/releases/2003/07/20030702-3.html*

[3] "Groups Join Experts in AIDS War," *The Nation*, September 22, 2003.

[4] **Nakazibwe, Carolyne (2003)**, "Country Leads in AIDS 'Care'," "The *Monitor*, September 23.

[5] "Traditional Healers Demand Recognition in Battle Against AIDS," Africa Church Information Service, September 25, 2003.

[6] "Male Machismo a Setback in the Fight Against HIV," *New Vision* (Uganda), September 30, 2003.

[7] **Bakyawa, Jennifer, (2003)**, "Women Hold the Key in AIDS Fight—Kibaki," *The Monitor* (Uganda), September 23.

[8] "Women Alone Can't Stop AIDS in Africa," *The East African Standard*,

September 28, 2003.

[9] **Mulumba, Badru (2003),** "First Lady Cautions on Use of Condoms," *The Monitor,* October 3.

[10] **Kinyungu, Cyrus (2003),** "More HIV Infections Blamed on Needles, Syringes," *The East African,* October 6-12, p.4.

[11] **Kimani, Dagi (2003a),** "Aids: Now Kenya Awards Tenders For ARVs...," *The East African,* October 6-12, p. 6.

[12] **Kwayera, Juma (2003),** "... As Losing CD4 Bidder Cries Foul," *The East African,* October 6-12, p. 6.

[13] **Clarey, Christopher (2003),** "Sports Stars Must Shine Brighter in Aids Fight," *The East African,* October 6-12, p.38.

[14] **Johnstone, Ralph (2003),** "Sex and Aids in Africa: Kibera Groups Offer Shocking Insights," *The East African,* October 6-12, Part 2, p. VII.

[15] **Wanyeki, L. Muthoni (2003),** "Aids: What Kibaki Should Tell Bush," *The East African,* October 6-12, p. 13.

[16] **Thomson, Alistair (2003),** "S.Africa AIDS Activist Gets Nobel Peace Nomination," Reuters, December 2.

[17] **Kimani, Dagi (2003b),** "Activists of the World, Chill Out, We've Heard You," *The East African,* October 6-12, p. 36.

[18] **Mwaura, Gitura (2003),** "Only the Activists Can Make Big Pharma Behave," *The East African,* October 13-19.

7

AIDS in African Fiction:
Imagination in the African AIDS Discourse

We have traveled some distance from the opening chapter. We began with an apparently sensible altruistic offer of $15 billion from America to address the problem of AIDS in Africa in 2003. The offer came as publicity about AIDS in Africa increased; it also came on the heels of the discovery that there was *something* we could do for people infected with HIV — that is, ARVs. It was, in addition, a surprise, coming as it did from a Republican administration, and it received support from liberals and conservatives alike.

Yet as we saw in the last chapter, Africans viewed the Western approach to the epidemic, represented by the US plan, with muted enthusiasm. What we have tried to show in all the chapters is that, first, there is a well-thought-out African understanding of this disease, and second, that this understanding differs substantially at some points from the Western approach. We can see some of the most subtle and nuanced differences in fiction.

Fictions are stories that are untrue, yet fiction is often anything but untrue. In Phaswane Mpe's 2001 novel *Welcome To Our Hillbrow*, the narrator is talking to the main character Refentse who has written a short story: "Euphemism. Xenophobia. Prejudice. AIDS. You wrote your story to think through all these issues, child of Tiragalong and Hillbrow."[1] Refentse, like Mpe and dozens of other novelists in Africa, needed to "think through all these issues", and found fiction the best way to do this. These are complex matters. AIDS is only one of many problems that trouble Africans; other novelists have added poverty, unemployment, sexism, culture, war, hypocrisy and so many other "issues" to the narrator's list. And the complexity does not just come from the "issues" themselves: many Africans have important relationships to both their home village and major urban centers, and are truly children of Tiragalong (the village) and Hillbrow (the city). Could the sciences ever be big enough to explore all of this? Isn't this complex situation precisely where we need to hear what comes from the imagination of African artists?

In this chapter we will look in detail at one African novel in which AIDS (the "last plague") is the main character. Then we will consider some of the themes referred to in both this novel and in several other works of African fiction, most published only in Africa, to see how they contribute to the African discourse of AIDS. This final chapter also serves as a recapitulation of many of the themes which have appeared throughout this book.

The Last Plague

Meja Mwangi's *The Last Plague*[2] takes place in the mythical village of Crossroads in an unnamed African country — probably Kenya. "Crossroads was dying; any old fool could see that." In the opening chapter the daily bus rolls into the sleepy dusty village, discharging three people and their baggage: two huge cartons and a coffin. An old couple are bringing home their son, who has died of Aids; the woman is Janet, our main character, who is bringing in cartons of condoms.

By 2000, when this book was published, Aids had already lost its capital letters in much of Africa. Like radar and scuba diving in the West, it had ceased being an acronym. It was no longer the Acquired Immune Deficiency Syndrome described by American and French doctors, attacking homosexual men and intravenous drug users. It was simply Aids, a plague that seemed to be attacking everyone in Africa. Joseph Situma titled his AIDS novel *The Mysterious Killer*[3] — but it was set in the 1980s and early 90s. By the time of Mwangi's novel, the disease was less mysterious, though still a puzzle to some. The old couple here are not sure why their son died; they are simply grieving.

But for Janet, "the condom woman," there is no mystery to the disease at all; part of her job is to clarify that it is simply a disease, not a curse from God, and that it has causes that can be identified and prevented. Her frustration is that the people in her village, she feels, do not listen to reason and do not take steps to prevent the disease. The question for Janet — and presumably for the author — is not whether or not a virus causes the disease, nor where that virus comes from. Janet does not think witchcraft causes Aids, even though she is working in a very traditional culture. However, she knows which of those traditional cultural practices contributes to Aids and, as we shall see, fights against them. She also has no doubt that unequal gender roles contribute to the epidemic. She is well aware of the subordinate role of women in African society, and does not like it. But she does not let that role keep her from doing what she thinks is necessary to control the plague.

Early in the *Plague* story, 27 year old Frank comes back home to Crossroads, presumably from the capital city—and everyone knows something is wrong. He is thin and sad and looks wretched. And, we discover, he did not go abroad to school as everyone in the village assumed he would. We eventually find out that he had received a positive HIV test, and had come home to die. However, Janet is not ready to let anyone just die. For her, the non-mysterious plague is marching on, and she wants help fighting it—including Frank's help.

Janet's sister Julia is married to Kata Kataa, a traditional healer and the chief circumciser in the village. His brother Pastor Solomon has just died of Aids, and in traditional African culture he (Kata) would inherit Solomon's wife—to help her financially and bear children for his brother. Janet understands that Solomon had likely already infected his wife, who would then infect Kata and consequently her sister Julia. To protect her sister from getting Aids, she decides that Kata must not take Solomon's wife as his second wife. She tells Julia. Julia protests that she cannot go against the culture, at which point their grandmother joins the discussion and accuses Janet of trying to change their traditions. Janet responds that she has no wish to change their customs – the plague, she says, will do that.

Since Julia does not feel comfortable talking with Kata, Janet asks Frank, as another man, to do so. He initially refuses, but Janet "persuades" him: she has a small piece of land he needs to build an animal clinic (he had studied veterinary medicine), and she agrees to lease it to him only if he agrees to talk with Kata. He does—with disastrous results. Kata throws him out of his compound and tries to kill him.

Modifying culture is never easy. But Janet continues to buck the culture head-on, and continues to lose. Every day she talks to people in her village about condoms and family planning and the risks of sexually transmitted diseases, and every day people run and hide when they see her coming. She is a campaigner, an activist who knows she is right, and the hostile reception she often receives only reinforces her conviction to continue. She even becomes involved in a poster campaign which employs inappropriately explicit illustrations (according to the villagers) – but she does not question their appropriateness. The job, for her, is literally a matter of life and death.

Since Frank failed to change Kata's mind, she continues to pursue the matter alone. She sues Kata, and brings the case to the local village court. Uncle Mark, one of the enigmatic old men in the village, surprisingly agrees with Janet, saying that Kata should not marry Solomon's wife since he died of the plague. Kata's response to them unravels the hearing. He announces that his brother died from witchcraft, not Aids. A young man in the crowd heckles him for suggesting this, and Kata attack the man, precipitating a general riot – and no conclusion to Janet's suit.

But Janet is not finished. When she finds out that Kata (Swahili for "cut") is about to perform the usual mass circumcision on the young men of the village, she attends — and this time Frank comes. It is of course inappropriate for a woman to attend the circumcision ritual, but her concern, again, is not cultural appropriateness, but the health of the people of Crossroads. Since the ritual is carried out with a single knife, she proclaims to the boys that if one of them has Aids, they will all get it and die. Once again, chaos ensues, this time with an attack on Frank, who dared to accompany Janet. He is chased by a mob of circumcisers and circumcisees, and once again just barely escapes.

This time he has had enough, and decides to leave Crossroads. Unfortunately for him, Janet is on the same bus out, carrying condoms and birth control pills to the next village. She chooses a seat next to him and begins her pitch to convince him to stay and help her fight Aids. She reminds him of the orphanage they had planned for Aids orphans. When Frank suggests that their mothers or other women should take care of them, Janet becomes angry, and begins a diatribe against selfish men. They get the opportunities to go abroad, she says, leaving the work of raising their children to their wives. The conversation spreads to the other passengers on the bus – at least the other women. The men keep very quiet.

When they arrive at the village, Frank helps Janet unload her supplies. An old woman who recognizes Janet asks why she is still telling people not to have babies, even though so many people are dying. Janet says she sees no reason to have babies today, only to bury them tomorrow. The old woman disagrees: having babies, she says, is God's way; it is a woman's fate. Janet will have none of this, and tells her so: women, she says, should have children by choice. At this the old woman can only laugh. "Go tell that to the men," she says.

Janet, still looking for a way to convince Frank to stay, makes it clear to those gathered around her that he is an animal doctor—and they immediately seek his advice and boost his ego. A short time later, she again presents him with the urgency of the task confronting her, and hopefully him as well. In an attempt to get away he pulls out what he feels is his trump card, that he is dying. Janet is not impressed – everyone is dying, she says. Frank struggles to explain that his situation is different, but Janet tells him she already knows why he came back, even though he had not told anyone. No one, she says, returns to Crossroads, a place with no secrets, except to die. Frank realizes he no longer has a secret, is relieved, and decides he can die in peace. Janet sees it differently: he can now, she says, live in hope, and with a purpose, and commit himself to her work. Frank is convinced, and stays in Crossroads.

More than one third of the way through the book, we meet Broker, who arrives, like so many other sleazy untrustworthies in African fiction, in a big car, black, with silver trimmings and tinted windows. Broker is in every sense an untrustworthy broker, and now he is also broken. He is emaciated, his hair is thin, his ears too large, and his eyes lost in their sockets. Yet despite his physical wasting, he is obviously rich. He is dressed in a flashy suit, big black shoes, and has a gold watch which hangs loosely from his bony wrist.

Broker is also returning home to die. He has gotten Aids during ten years of fast and loose urban living. He had left Crossroads with a woman who wasn't his wife, and now expects to return to his wife, Janet. Not surprisingly, she wants nothing to do with him. Janet also gets pressure from her grandmother to take him back, but she is steadfast. Broker may have been her husband before, but, she tells him, he lost that right.

But though he is dying, he has not stopped being a broker. While he continues to try to wheedle his way back into Janet's home, he also tries to go into business. He spends the rest of the book trying to pick up the pieces of his broken life, but also trying to broker the rejuvenation of the Crossroads economy (finally rebuilding a gas station!). As part of that rebuilding, he eventually makes his own contribution to Janet's condom campaign.

But not right away; it takes a while before Janet can hear him. The condom campaign is not in fact going well, but Janet just wants to do more of the same. Frank suggests that people don't use condoms because they don't value them; one way to give them value is to make people pay for them. Janet refuses: they are government condoms, she says, and they are supposed to be free. But before they have a chance to further debate the merits of selling vs. giving, they are both summonsed to court for corrupting the morals of the youth with their condom distribution and poster campaign.

The case is no more conclusive than when Janet sued Kata. Uncle Mark, the same old man who sided with Janet in that suit, concludes this case also. He suggests that the Chief tell the people that their survival does not depend on the government, nor on condoms from foreigners, but "that our health and that of our community depends on us, ourselves." The Chief says he is not authorized to do that. Uncle Mark suggests, then, that the chief simply tell the villagers to go to hell – but he responds that he is not authorized to do that either. The case almost ends in a stalemate again, but Frank and Janet are finally given begrudging permission to proceed quietly with their campaign.

Broker now decides it's time for his contribution. He presents himself to Janet and Frank, and declares, after a long exhausting introduction, that the way to make people understand the epidemic and accept the condom is to sell it. Exasperated—and worn down—Janet gives him one carton of condoms to sell. Broker then brings all of the big city business skills that made him rich to the task of selling condoms. When people tell him that condoms are free, he brings them up to date: "There's nothing for free anymore; this is the new world order." He goes to a general store to try and persuade the proprietor to carry condoms in his store.

> The trader took the condom and examined it curiously. Like many people in Crossroads, he had never before seen a condom at such close quarters, and was now surprised to see how simple and ordinary it looked.
>
> "But do not underrate this little bit of latex," Broker warned him. "The only thing it will not do is sing *Happy Birthday To You*."...
>
> The trader scrutinized the condom, glanced again over his shoulder and finally asked, "How does it work?"
>
> "How does what work?" Broker asked him.
>
> "*Kodom*," said the man.
>
> "How does a condom work?" Broker asked, confused. "What do you mean how does a condom work?"
>
> "Does it have batteries?" asked the man.
>
> "What for does it need batteries?" Broker asked.
>
> "You say this *thing* can sing," said the man.
>
> "Did I say that?" Broker was devastated. "No, I did not say that."[4]

Despite this slow start, he eventually manages to sell all the condoms in the carton, he tells Janet, and now wants to expand the business. He wants to open a condom shop. Janet is nonplussed; Broker promises to use all the proceeds to support Aids orphans. Janet thinks it's a crazy idea; she worries and worries, and somehow agrees.

In spite of her worries, the activities around the Condom Shop, together with Janet's persistent community education, eventually attract the attention of even those outside of Crossroads—including the government Ministry of Health. They send Janet a letter (which she receives three months later!) informing her of an upcoming visit from some officials of an international commission that has heard of her work in the community, and want to see it first-hand. Janet and her co-workers are intrigued, but the part of the letter that generates the most discussion among them is the promise of anything she needs; all that's required is that she ask. Her co-workers develop a remarkable list in a very short time: a video machine, a farm, money, a water tank, a clinic, a car, a well, a radio, a bicycle... But Janet has other ideas.

Then one day, without warning, she gets a message that the Chief wants to see her, together with several other government officials and the white men from the international commission. She worries aloud that they will find their free condoms being sold — but Broker tells her to go meet the team, and he will take care of everything with the shop.

When she arrives at the Chief's office, she is naturally nervous, especially with so many white people. They introduce themselves quickly and then the leader, Don Donovan – who does most of the talking and asks few questions – announces that they are very interested in Janet's work, but have little time to see it. Nevertheless, he asks her to show them everything that she's been doing – in three hours.

Throughout the visit, the visitors and villagers each play their roles flawlessly, the visitors uncovering the "right" issues, and the villagers giving the "right" answers—though sometimes Janet needs to prompt them in their local language. They begin at the school, where the team is impressed by and photographs the posters that the villagers felt were inappropriately explicit. One journalist notes the "environmental pollution" (the ubiquitous plastic bags blowing in the wind) and asks a villager where they dispose of used condoms. The villager is stumped, but Janet rescues him and says that all used condoms go in the latrines, not the household compost piles. Don Donovan is impressed with this "right answer".

They next move to the church where Janet and Frank had hoped to develop the orphanage. Janet tells the pastor they have come to see his work on behalf of the orphans. The pastor is unaware of the work he is doing until Janet informs him.

Eventually they meet Broker who offers to show them the Condom Clinic – he had painted over the word *Shop* and had scrawled in its place *Clinic*. The video cameraman asks him to organize a queue of people lining up for the *free* condoms, which Broker himself joins. The journalist asks him why he needs condoms and he explains that though he is HIV positive, he is still sexually very active and wants to protect his partner who he loves very much. Most people, he continues, don't understand that even with Aids it is possible to continue an active sex life, and he explains how. He talks so long, in fact, that the cameraman runs out of tape.

At the end of the visit, Don Donovan asks Janet if there is anything she needs from them, but before she can answer, Broker says they need a vehicle. It takes a while before Janet finally gets the discussion back on *her* track, but she eventually does. What she wants, she says, more than a car or anything else, is to have free Aids tests for all the people in Crossroads.

Previously, when the letter had first come and everyone was making a wish list, Janet had told them the same thing: she wanted to know how many people were *free* from Aids. They wanted to know why that was important. She had told them that despair and ignorance were the biggest problems she encountered in her fight against Aids. She said people who thought they might be infected would simply give up, and not even try to protect themselves or others. Knowing their status, she felt, would help them, and her, focus the fight against the plague.

The visit from the international commission ends satisfactorily for the visitors and for Janet, with Don Donovan agreeing to consider Janet's request; but the villagers are unhappy. They want to know where the presents are, the money that the visitors who came in all those cars had brought for them. They wait around in a crowd, but when no presents appear, they disperse, no better off than before the visitors came.

Several months later another Ministry of Health team arrives, unannounced, to do the survey Janet had asked for. Some villagers agree to be tested, but the majority are skeptical, seeing the exercise as a research project, one that they want no part of. But, says the European advisor, the small sample they did test was good enough for generating statistics. The team leaves, and the villagers are left to mull over what a positive test would mean.

Frank and Broker walk together by the once mighty village river that had become only a sickly, slimy stream because of deforestation. Frank admits to Broker that he is HIV positive, something Broker had already figured out. After a pause, Broker asks how he found out. It was just a routine check-up, Frank tells him, but the positive test means he lost his scholarship and the rest of his education. Broker says he was sick when he was tested, and was devastated by the result. Frank says he thought of suicide; Broker says he couldn't think at all.

Weeks later the convoy of vehicles returns to Crossroads with another team to distribute the HIV test results. Some people come out of the office screaming, some dancing; one woman simply faints. Big Youth, a faithful but simple colleague of Janet, not understanding his results, asks Frank:

> "What does it mean HIV minus?"
> "It means HIV negative," Frank replied.
> "Is it good news or bad news?" he asked.
> "The best news you ever prayed for," Broker told him.
> "Does it mean I don't have Aids?" his voice rose a notch.
> "That's right," Frank told him. "You don't have Aids."[5]

Julia, Janet's sister, also gets her test result, and it too is negative. But she doesn't simply rejoice; she decides that the only way she can be sure to stay negative is to stop having sex with her husband Kata. He had previously begrudgingly agreed to use condoms and not sleep with his dead brother's wife after looking through a particularly gruesome medical textbook that Janet had loaned to her. But Janet had warned her then that although

150

condoms were better than nothing, only total abstinence was completely safe.

Just after Julia gets her report, Frank gets his—and it too is negative. It turns out that for several years Frank has been living with a false positive result. He lost a chance to go abroad to study, almost killed himself, and came home to die—all because of a blood test that was inaccurate.

Nevertheless, despite the hope that these several negative tests point to at the end of the story, Aids still kills. Even Broker cannot broker a deal that will keep him from dying. Shortly before his death, he and Janet go back into the woods where they used to wander as young lovers.

> Just as Aids had deprived the valley of its life, the loggers had deprived the hills of their cover, leaving them grotesquely naked and vulnerable to the vagaries of the weather. Where once they had been shrouded in mystery and the promise of romantic adventure, the hills were now plain and bare with nothing to offer an intrepid heart....
>
> ... The old brook was a sickly grey stream and the grass along its banks was coarse and dry from exposure. The ebony tree under which her son was conceived was long gone, murdered in its prime to make wood for the coffins, and in its place sat an impenetrably thorny bush, thick and useless....[6]

External environmental devastation mirrors the internal immune deficiency. Something is cosmically wrong.

THEMES

The Last Plague is long enough for Mwangi to uncover several themes or issues, hints at what might be cosmically wrong. These same themes appear in other shorter novels by African writers, and not surprisingly mirror the issues that we have been considering in this book. While some of the novels are more obviously written to inform and to warn, such as *Confessions of an AIDS Victim*[7], others intend more to explore, or even just expose the social and emotional terrain of AIDS in Africa. Nevertheless, several themes reoccur in these varied stories.

GENDER

Of the novels and stories I read, nearly half were written by women, and in the majority of all of them the main character is a woman. Prof Nobantu Rasebotsa in Botswana provides an excellent analysis of gender issues in four of these novels[8]; here I merely want to highlight the issue.

In the first paragraph of *The Plague At My Door* we meet Tamara, "a lawyer and well-known advocate of women's rights. She often complained that African women had 'a raw deal both in their homes and in the country.'... Her main interest was trying to improve the situation of women in the country, who, she felt, were being discriminated against. She believed that unless women were give equal opportunities in all spheres of life, the country would lag behind in development." One day her husband invites her to go on a business trip with him, "but she had refused, telling him that she was too busy and that her career was as important as his."[9] He is depressed, he drinks too much, has a single encounter with a prostitute, and becomes infected with AIDS. He eventually tells his wife and accepts responsibility for his mistake. She fortunately is not infected because due to "problems with other contraceptives" they had been using condoms.

In this novella, written by a Zambian woman author, four other characters get AIDS—one is a traveling salesman with several girlfriends, who brings AIDS home and infects his wife, and the other two are women who get accidentally infected, one by a needle-stick and the other by a blood transfusion. Clearly women are the victims—at least in this story. In some of the other novels the gender focus is presented more subtly, but no less firmly:

The main character Mosa in Unity Dow's *Far and Beyon'*, as a teenager, "was quickly accepting the special place of men in her society. They were responsible for very little. If she wanted to go far and beyon', she would have to start with accepting that basic reality."[10] She does, and goes "beyon'" it. Rachel, the main character in *The Mysterious Killer*, would prefer to ignore that reality, and acts as though there are no gender expectations placed on her. She is also an activist. This combination—ignoring gender expectations and activism—gets her in trouble, as we will see. Janet had already accepted the "basic reality" of men's irresponsibility long before *The Last Plague* opens. But for none of these women does accepting that basic reality mean submitting to it. They all decide to do something about Aids in their communities. The only men I found who were "activists" against Aids were a medical researcher in *Deadly Profit*[11] and a doctor specializing in sexually transmitted diseases in *Nice People*[12]

But there are other female characters who are not activists, who simply try to live with their diagnosis. Catherine Njeri, the narrator and main character in *Confessions of an AIDS Victim*, tells her story almost clinically, and the straightforward account of her infection is demystifying. She is clear where she was deceived by a man; she is also clear in accepting her own responsibility. In two other novels, women make personal choices that show their individual strength: Ttiisa in *Vanishing Shadows*[13] chooses not to be sexually active following the apparent AIDS-related death of her young husband and infant son, and Loveness in *Waste Not Your Tears*[14] eventually leaves her lover who has deliberately infected her.

CHURCH

In *The Last Plague*, Kata Kataa is supposed to inherit his brother's wife after his brother dies of Aids. His brother is *Pastor* Solomon. Clearly the church provided no protection against him getting infected. The church does not fare well generally in this book. When the visitors come to see Janet's anti-Aids work, she has to prompt another pastor to give the right answer about the orphanage being built at his church. The reason for the prompting is that he had previously opposed its development. His "parish committee was composed of a motley group of old men and women; a self-satisfied group to whom the crumbling old church was their only refuge, a private ground where only the chosen and the privileged had a right to be." The first time the orphanage was voted down, the pastor's influence was clear: "All those in favor of turning this hallowed ground into a playground for sin raise your hands."[15]

The church fares no better in *The Mysterious Killer*. Early in the story, Rachel, a resolute young woman, is influenced by the teaching and example of the priest, Father Michael. His sermons and energy are admirable, but neither enables him to resist the temptation he struggles with toward another young woman in the church. He is eventually transferred to another district—but is there confronted again with the young woman and her child, which is his child. Meanwhile, Rachel proceeds with her anti-AIDS activity outside the context of the church.

On the other hand, Loveness in *Waste Not Your Tears* finds in the church a source of strength. When she is acutely ill, a nun visits her in the hospital. She tells the story of how she has been abused by her lover, afraid that the nun will force her to return to him. But she finds instead comfort, and stays with the nuns for a while, who enable her to reconnect with her father—and not return to her lover.

Probably the most nuanced treatment of the church is in Marjorie Macgoye's *Chira*[16]. The author, born in England, came to Kenya in the 1950s as a missionary bookseller. She eventually married a Kenyan and became a Kenyan citizen. Where the church in *The Last Plague* is probably mainline Protestant, and in *Mysterious* and *Waste Not* is clearly Catholic, *Chira* introduces us to an independent store-front church in Nairobi. The pastor is young, sincere, and energetic—but still practical. The main character Otieno joins his church and finds there a source of strength and support in his not always successful attempts to avoid sexual activity before marriage. The church for him is at least a community of somewhat like-minded people—and a practical source of help for people when they are sick.

Otieno's theology, however, is more muddled. Concerning evil: "The best defense against the unthinkable was to deny it. Reality could be caged in a tight-woven basket of assertions; you smeared over the cracks with repetitions like cow-dung. Was that not what you did in church, joining so often with many voices in the creed that any doubt or contradiction was hedged inside?" Nor had he resolved the conflict with his ancestral beliefs: "Had you not better hedge your bet if all the ceremonies of wailing and recall have more force for you than the empty tomb?"[17] For Macgoye, the ex-missionary, it seems that the church still has a role to play in the fight against AIDS, even if that role is not a theological one.

There is a very different perspective of church—or rather of God—from a medical thriller written by a Zimbabwean doctor living in South Africa. Patrice Matchaba's *Deadly Profit* is mostly about the intrigues of pharmaceutical industry research, and his characters are all doctors (African), scientists (European), and financiers (American). The world they inhabit is very rich and very secular, and their church connections (if they have any) are never mentioned. But all of them, even the New York businesswoman, have a bedrock faith in God's presence and sovereignty.

The characters are aware of "God's plan" and the "journey God had set for us." One, a South African doctor, suggested that "what was needed wasn't a vaccine, but that Jesus would have to come again and teach us the value of love and sacrifice for one another." The same character, speaking about the New York businesswoman, says "In a sense it was as if she had now realized what God had also done through the death of his only son. This sacrifice was necessary for mankind to make progress and would be played out in different parts of the world every day."[18] This God-consciousness, or at least moral foundation, seems to influence their behavior as well. There are four couples in the novel, and none of them married—yet only one of these eight characters is unfaithful throughout the course of the novel.

ORPHANS

When Janet and Frank try to build an orphanage, they are met with opposition from an unsympathetic, moralizing pastor. The other novels are strangely silent about orphanages, and even about AIDS orphans—far more silent than the Western media. But Africa does not ignore AIDS orphans. Another novel from Kenya, though not

155

dealing directly with AIDS, gives us some insight into an African view.

In Margaret Ogola's *I Swear By Apollo*[19], the main characters are doctors with six of their own children, and three nieces and nephews who live with them because their parents died of AIDS. Though this stretches the "nuclear" family in the novel, the other children are welcome because of responsibility for the extended family. The author, in an interview, expands on this stretching: "AIDS has come at a time when our families have been very seriously weakened by aggressive population control that has been conducted in Africa for the last 40 years" meaning "there's just not enough people to 'pick up the pieces' to care for the orphans."[20] We in the West may want to defend our population control efforts, but we are obliged to listen to African opinion about these activities, as well as the negative side effects of shrinking extended families.

CULTURE

Traditional culture is clearly more potent in rural areas. Janet in rural Kenya was constantly encountering resistance to her attempts at education—resistance rooted in conservative cultural beliefs. It was the same with Rachel in her village in the fictitious country of Randi (Randi = randy, British slang for horny). In *The Mysterious Killer*, she convinces the elders of her village to declare a sex moratorium to try to control Aids—and later gets raped by opponents of this plan. Culture is also powerful in rural Botswana, but Mosa in *Far and Beyon'* takes a much gentler approach than either Rachel or Janet. She has lost two brothers to Aids, and watches her mother perform ritual after ritual to counteract the witchcraft she (the mother) believes caused their deaths. Mosa chooses to go along with the rituals she feels do no harm, but eventually works to reunite her mother with the woman—a former close friend—who the diviner said was the witch.

However, traditional culture is often diluted in African cities. It is still remembered—most city people have relatives in villages— but for novelists at least it is less of a force. Characters living in Nairobi (*Confessions of an AIDS Victim* and *Nice People*), Kampala

(*Vanishing Shadows*), Harare (*Waste Not Your Tears*), and Cape Town (*Deadly Profit*) don't have the same battles with culture that Janet and Rachel and Mosa do. In *Welcome To Our Hillbrow*, the characters live the urban life while they are in Johannesburg, but have to deal with the consequences when they go back to their home village. But of course all of these urban dwellers still face the risks of AIDS, and these "urban" novels paint a clear picture of a life of multiple sexual partners. In *Confessions*, *Deadly Profit*, *Nice People*, and *Hillbrow*, the characters, both male and female, are upwardly mobile, living "in the fast lane". But in *Waste Not Your Tears* (and likely in *Vanishing Shadows* as well) it is clearly the urban man who has multiple partners, and the woman who is the victim. Even in *Deadly Profit*, the novel least involved with traditional culture, one of the AIDS patients is a woman, infected with HIV by her very first lover.

CARS

In *The Last Plague*, we first meet Broker when he drives up in a big car. The car seems to symbolize wealth obtained illicitly, and hints at sex obtained illicitly. In *The Mysterious Killer*, Rachel's dying aunt "Cecilia returned, with her friend, who owned a Mercedes Benz...."[21] Cecilia is dying of AIDS. In *Nice People*, one of the nice people with AIDS drives to the clinic in a BMW; another, on finding his diagnosis, shoots himself in his Mercedes Benz. In *Confessions*, the narrator Catherine early on "noticed Henry seated in a cool blue Peugeot 504 saloon" car. She joins him, gets half-drunk, and loses her virginity: "He had told me to trust him as he would not go all the way and he mercilessly breached the trust."[22]

Yet without the car, there is no love—or at least no sex. In *Welcome To Our Hillbrow*, the central character Refentse's first love goes nowhere: "You simply loved the woman, who loved you back, but who was honest enough to tell you that although she loved you, she was not prepared to have a relationship with you because you did not have a car."[23]

But, as with sex, there is ambivalence about cars. The sign of economic development at the very end of *The Last Plague* is the rebirth of the service station in Crossroads, engineered by Broker.

WESTERN VIEWS/NGOs

The Last Plague provides us with the most extensive look at the interaction between Western organizational approaches to AIDS and how villagers respond. In some of the novels, these organizations are in the background; in others, we don't see them at all. But today, especially as more and more Western money is going to address African AIDS, it is important to see how Africans view this.

Janet promotes condoms and blood testing, two hallmarks of the Western approach. It seems that she believes passionately in both, though many in her village remain unconvinced by the end of the story. Several characters, especially Kata and Julia, do individually change their views, and a substantial minority in the village do agree to be tested. It is unclear how the author views Janet's campaign, though he provides no other characters with alternative plans (except in the giving vs. selling condoms debate).

But if we are not sure of how the author views Western *approaches*, we are clearer about how he views the Western *people* that bring those approaches. When the people "from the world, the world... something or other" come, "Don Donovan did most of the talking and asked few questions." The outsiders go away with little clue of what is really going on in Crossroads. It is true that Broker is deceptive, changing the sign from *Condom Shop* to *Condom Clinic*. But clearly the largest deception is what the visitors bring on themselves, limiting their visit to three hours when they need three years to begin to understand.

There is a similar self-deception by a Westerner in *Waste Not Your Tears*. Roderick (Loveness's lover) is selfish and promiscuous, and as a result of his drinking he loses his apartment and his job. He coincidently tests positive for HIV, and tells the people at the AIDS Welfare Center that his positive test has cost him his job and home. An American, Dr. Baker, believes him—he needs to believe him because he needs articulate locals to help him in his AIDS education campaign. Dr. Baker showers him with gifts and never realizes, until the end of the book, that he is being deceived by Roderick. (When he finally does realize, he tries to get Loveness to sue Roderick!)

The earliest novel addressing AIDS that I found, *Nice People* (1992), takes place before and during the beginnings of the AIDS outbreak, and consequently does not deal with Western NGOs. However, Western ideas clearly influence the main character. He is a Kenyan doctor specializing in all the sexually transmitted diseases that preceded AIDS, and feels that a "moral stance contributed towards the failure to eradicate VDs." He argues "that openness in views of venereal diseases could help in fighting its spread" by making it easier for people to seek and obtain curative treatment—which should be offered free or at minimal cost. Instead of advocating behavior change for his patients (or himself), he wants "to remove sex from the shackles of morality."

However, his approach has less relevance when AIDS appears: there is no cure, and the very activities he defended and participated in were those that contributed to the spread of AIDS: "I had coitus severally with the three women, who had done the same with three and more men who in turn had themselves been involved with others. I saw the picture similar to that of a spider-web that traps any flies that come into it and I knew we were all in the web."[24] His free treatment and open attitude approach—while in itself admirable—had no application for AIDS control in Kenya.

Western NGOs are in the background of *Vanishing Shadows,* but by the end of the book become very important—not because they prevent AIDS, but because they are a source of employment for the two main characters. Throughout the book the driving passion for both of them is not avoiding AIDS, but finding work. For Africans in poor economies, this role of NGO as employer may be more important than what the NGOs offer in goods or services. As the role of outside money in AIDS care increases in Africa, it will be interesting to see how African novelists will view NGOs that bring ARV drug therapy, and how they will view the patients on this therapy.

DRUG TREATMENT

The one novel which touches on ARV drug treatment is *Deadly Profit*, though with a recognition that "the drugs were extremely expensive and... those in the developing countries... could never afford them." The title of this South African-published book (which ironically costs $200 used in the US, but only $15 new in UK) refers to the reluctance of the pharmaceutical companies to pursue vaccine research: "None of them were interested in vaccine research and it was no secret that they were making more money treating AIDS with the various drug cocktails..." The story contains Wall Street shenanigans involving even a US senator who "was using his political influence on Capitol Hill to get only the bills he wanted passed—those that would benefit him financially." [25]

Written in the later years of the Clinton presidency, the novel is troublingly prescient—except that there is nothing secretive or illegal in what the next administration did. As we have seen, President Bush upstaged his Democratic foes as well as the South African debate by offering $15 billion over five years to fight AIDS in Africa. We then saw that he chose a pharmaceutical company ex-CEO to head his program. By early 2004, generic drug combinations approved by the WHO —and made by Indian and other non-US companies—were available at one fourth of the cost of even the discounted brand-name drugs. However, the administration balked at buying these drugs.[26] It was hard to escape the conclusion that the US wanted its "aid" to go to its own companies, even if that meant treating only one fourth the number of people.

This theme of profit from the epidemic is also present in *Nice People*. Shortly after AIDS appears in Kenya, a private profit-driven hospital tries to cash in on the fear by regularly testing high-class prostitutes and selling certificates (of their sero-negativity) to them for rapidly increasing fees. The hospital's defense: "Oh! Who is not exploiting people through AIDS? The rubber manufacturers of America are making billions out of condoms.... Writers and film-makers are busy making hay when the sun shines with the AIDS scare. We must hurry.... We could make millions and each retire comfortably by the time they discover the cure." Will future novels see ARV drugs as that "cure", or as simply another chance "to cash in on the killer disease so long as people were so scared as to want" them?[27]

SUICIDE

Suicide looms large as a sub-plot in the Aids story. When Frank first got his positive Aids test, all he could think of was suicide, he tells Broker. Two characters in *Welcome To Our Hillbrow* take their own lives—not directly because of Aids, but as part of the confusing overlapping rural/urban, traditional/modern life that helps produce Aids in Africa today. One of these people has written a short story in which there is a young woman with AIDS. From the point of view of those in her village, "she was a child who had, in effect, committed suicide."[28] In *Vanishing Shadows*, when Ttiisa leaves her boyfriend a note that she has AIDS and then disappears, he immediately assumes she is considering suicide. When one character is told his diagnosis in *Nice People*, he "refused treatment at the Canaan Hospice and shot himself inside his Mercedes Benz."[29] Another character in the same book, on hearing her diagnosis, blows herself up in her Mercedes. The American woman in *Deadly Profit* tries to hang herself when she thinks she might be infected. In *The Mysterious Killer*, the priest who had originally inspired Rachel does hang himself because he believes he has been infected with HIV—believes for good reason, though he never took a test. And Rachel herself, after being tested because she had been raped, and getting a positive result, writes suicide notes and throws herself in front of a speeding minibus.

All cultures take suicide seriously, but it has a particularly disturbing meaning in Africa: "Victims of suicide are until today seen as witches in many African communities..."[30] Killing is bad in any society, but its connection with witchcraft magnifies its abhorrence. That so many people in these novels would attempt or commit suicide is surprising, reflecting both the hopelessness that the diagnosis raises, as well as the stigma that is attached to it.

FALSE POSITIVES

Frank's test, it turns out, was a false positive. But it's not only Frank. Rachel somehow survives her collision with the minibus, as well as her *false* positive HIV test: she is retested in the hospital and the test comes back negative. Mosa in *Far and Beyon'*, though having never been tested, is held hostage through most of the book to what her test might show—she had been pregnant but had an abortion. Her test too, in the last chapter, comes back negative. And Ttiisa from *Vanishing Shadows*—the one who wrote the note to her boyfriend and disappeared—had good reason to suspect AIDS: her lover had died rather suddenly, as had her infant son. But she too has had a "false positive diagnosis": when she is finally tested, the test is HIV negative.

Skeptics may interpret these many false positive diagnoses as a form of denial—mirroring, they might say, the official governmental denials they saw in the 1990s in many African countries. That is certainly one interpretation, but it risks not seeing what these novelists might be saying. A more obvious interpretation is that there *are* many false positive tests, as we saw in the chapter on the *New African*. We in the West may think false positive tests are no big deal, a fortunate mistake. We may or may not admit that excess false positives do make statistics look worse, increasing attention to African AIDS and funding for research and AIDS programs. But Africans do not necessarily see these latter as advantages: increased attention often only means increased pity, and false positive tests can destroy a person's life, as we saw with Frank.

AIDS KILLS

But clearly there is no denial of the real dangers of AIDS in these novels. Broker dies—along with someone else in Crossroads almost every day. In *Deadly Profit* "there was a funeral every other week... Soon there would be no space left to bury the dead..."[31] *Nice People* opens with the funeral of a young woman who has died of AIDS, and then flashes back to the events leading to her infection. Mosa's two brothers are dead at the beginning of *Far and Beyon'*. Rachel's aunt and those she overlapped with all die. Catherine ends her *Confessions* being "not happy at all, every minute I remember I am on the victims list and that I face the death penalty."[32] The two main characters in *Waste Not Your Tears* clearly have AIDS. Refilwe at the end of *Welcome To Our Hillbrow* is thin and sick with AIDS, almost ready to join in death those who have taken their own lives. And in "Effortless Tears"[33] we stand around the grave of George Pasi who has just died of AIDS. AIDS kills.

ENVIRONMENT

At the end of *The Last Plague* we saw how external environmental devastation was mirroring the internal immune deficiency. This theme permeates Alexander Kanengoni's short story "Effortless Tears" as well. The narrator's cousin George is dying of Aids.

> ... January's scorching sun in the naked sky and the suffocating air intensified into a sense of looming crisis that could not be expressed in words. The rains were already very late and the frequent sight of untilled fields, helplessly confronting an unfulfilling sky created images of seasons that could no longer be understood. The crops that had been planted with the first and only rains of the season had emerged only to fight a relentless war with the sun. Most had wilted and died. The few plants that still survived were struggling in the stifling heat.

At the burial,

> ... lean cattle, their bones sticking out, their ribs moving painfully under their taut skin, nibbled at something on the dry ground: what it was no one could make out. And around the grave the atmosphere was subdued and silent. Even the once phenomenal Save River, only a stone's throw away to the east, lay silent. This gigantic river, reduced to puddles between heaps of sand seemed to be brooding on its sad predicament... [34]

African fiction is not generally nihilistic, and none of these works are. Several show characters who have small victories in their attempts to slow the spread of AIDS, characters who end up *without* AIDS. Even the main character in *Nice People*, who has had frequent sex with three women, all of whom have or might have AIDS, is HIV negative. Rather than representing denial, this could reflect the hope which characterizes so much of African life.

But African fiction is also not generally a diversion, a pure entertainment, an escape. Something *is* wrong—not meaningless, but wrong—and what is wrong is not just wrong inside Africa. Matchaba, in a non-fiction Afterword to his novel, says, "It is ironic that the continent that has been hardest hit by AIDS has not only embraced the 'free market', but has also contributed much to the North's development, in terms of manpower and natural resources... [A]re we to believe that, because [AIDS is] not a major threat to people in the North, they are willing to watch as it decimates us in the South? Surely globalization must mean more than the South simply buying goods from the North. What has happened to our common goals and destiny as humans?"[35]

The context of these comments, admittedly, is a plea for market forces and technology to join in a fight against African AIDS. But it is hard, reading this quote, to escape the conclusion that something has gone horribly wrong with globalization. The internal immune deficiency mirrored by the external environmental devastation is mirrored yet again in global economic dominance and exploitation. Mirrored, not explained. These are novels, filled with suggestions, events, and metaphors. They are not trying to lay blame or prove anything or analyze AIDS, much less solve the problem. They are stories "to think through all these issues"—at most. But, as with all art, they can point beyond where we usually look. African imagination in fiction can not only enliven the discourse of AIDS in Africa, it can also help us to enter the mystery of what might be wrong—not only in Africa, but also in us.

REFERENCES

[1] **Mpe, Phaswane (2001),** *Welcome To Our Hillbrow* (Pietermaritzburg, University of Natal Press), p.60.

[2] **Mwangi, Meja (2000),** *The Last Plague* (Nairobi, East African Educational Publishers).

[3] **Situma, Joseph (2001),** *The Mysterious Killer* (Nairobi, Africawide Network).

[4] **Mwangi,** *op. cit.,* **2000,** p. 257.

[5] **Mwangi,** *op. cit.,* **2000,** p. 415.

[6] **Mwangi,** *op. cit.,* **2000,** p. 443.

[7] **Adalla, Carolyne (1993),** *Confessions of an AIDS Victim* (Nairobi, Spear Books).

[8] **Rasebotsa, Nobantu (2004),** "AIDS Fiction in Africa" in *The Discourse of Hiv/Aids in Africa* edited by E Biakolo, J Mathangwane, and D Odallo (Pretoria and Gabarone, UNAIDS).

[9] **Nyaywa, Kekelwa (1996),** *The Plague At My Door* (Randburg, South Africa, Ravan Press), p. 1, 43-4, 65..

[10] **Dow, Unity (2000),** *Far and Beyon'* (Gaborone, Longman), p. 76.

[11] **Matchaba, Patrice (2000),** *Deadly Profit* (Capetown, David Philip Publishers).

[12] **Geteria, Wamugunda (1992),** *Nice People* (Nairobi, East African Educational Publishers).

[13] **Kayondo, Namige (1995),** *Vanishing Shadows* (Oxford, Macmillan).

[14] **Kala, Violet (1994),** *Waste Not Your Tears* (Harare, Baobab Books).

[15] **Mwangi,** *op. cit.,* **2000,** p. 121-2.

[16] **Macgoye, Marjorie (1997),** *Chira* (Nairobi, East African Educational Publishers).

[17] **Macgoye,** *Ibid.,* **1997,** p. 45, 61.

[18] **Matchaba,** *op. cit.,* **2000,** p. 24-5, 34, 151.

[19] **Ogola, Margaret (2002),** *I Swear By Apollo* (Nairobi, Focus Books).

[20] **Ogola, Margaret (1999),** in "Interview with Dr. Margaret Ogola of Kenya—'Condom Use Spread AIDS'", Nov 18, 1999, *www.bannerofliberty.com/BOL-03MQC/1-31-2003.2.html*

[21] **Situma,** *op. cit.,* **2001,** p. 28.

[22] **Adalla,** *op. cit.,* **1993,** p. 25, 28-9.

[23] **Mpe,** *op. cit.,* **2001,** p. 88.

[24] **Geteria,** *op. cit.,* **1992,** p. 77, 109, 78, 167.

[25] **Matchaba,** *op. cit.,* **2000,** p. 71-2.

[26] "8,000 Deaths a Day," Editorial, *The Washington Post*, March 26, 2004, p. A22.

[27] **Geteria,** *op. cit.,* **1992,** p. 170-1, 169.

[28] **Mpe,** *op. cit.,* **2001,** p. 54.

[29] **Geteria,** *op. cit.,* **1992,** p. 162.

[30] **Magesa, Laurenti (2000),** "Recognizing the Reality of African Religion in Tanzania," in *Catholic Ethicists on HIV/AIDS Prevention* edited by James F. Keenan et al (New York, Continuum), p. 82.

[31] **Matchaba,** *op. cit.,* **2000,** p. 58-9.

[32] **Adalla,** *op. cit.,* **1993,** p. 82.

---

[33] **Kanengoni, Alexander (1993),** "Effortless Tears" in *Effortless Tears* (Harare, Baobab Books).

[34] **Kanengoni,** *Ibid.,* **1993**, p. 72-3.

[35] **Matchaba,** *op. cit.,* **2000**, p. 179.

Afterword:
Ways of Living

There is one more thing.

What do we do, what does Africa do, when more and more people die from AIDS, when prevention stalls, when treatment is not available? Africa—the continent of incomprehensible hope, the place of "life in all its fullness"—mourns.

Meet Toloki, the Professional Mourner, the main character in Zakes Mda's *Ways of Dying*. It is South Africa, just before their first free election. In the political violence, people are dying more than they used to. Middle aged and young people are dying—people that don't usually seem to die. A woman who has lost her brother goes to the morgue to try and find him. There she finds 20 naked bodies on the floor, "all victims of the raging war consuming our lives."[1] It could have been AIDS. Funerals used to be just on the weekends, but now there are too many—several every day, even simultaneously in the same cemetery. Toloki has come from the village to the city *to make a life* but it is hard. Things don't work. A furniture maker from his village, also living in the city, has discovered a way to make a living from death: he makes coffins. In fact, he becomes very rich. This gives Toloki the idea to begin the profession of Professional Mourner.

He obtains a uniform—a top-hat, a black silk cape, and black trousers—and begins going to funerals, sitting on the pile of dirt next to the freshly dug grave, weeping. Sometimes he weeps quietly; sometimes he invents new heart-breaking sounds. He expects to be paid for his work, and he is, mostly at the funerals of poor people. They, at least, appreciate that he cares enough to mourn.

His understanding of his role gradually changes and grows. He begins mourning as a job, but comes to realize it as a calling. He finds out about ascetic Hindu monks, and begins to fashion himself after them. When his squatter shack is torched, he moves to a waiting room beside a wharf in the harbor, with all of his belongings stored in a shopping cart. He looks like a crazy homeless bum—but he understands his mourning as a "spiritual vocation": he mourns for the nation.

On Christmas day, Toloki attends the funeral of a child, and listens to how he died: "'There are many ways of dying!...This our brother's way is a way that has left us without words in our mouths. This little brother was our own child, and his death is more painful because it is of our own creation.'"[2] Could this be a story about AIDS? Toloki eventually meets the mother of the child who has died—a woman, it turns out, from his home village. He has not seen her since childhood; now he is 38, she is 35. During the week between Christmas and New Years, they reconnect.

She has had a hard life, and though only 35, "has grown old now, and has become a little haggard. But she is still beautiful."[3] Noria is her name. She had always been liberal sharing her beauty with men—too liberal. She ran away with a teenage boy and had a child—but both her child and husband died. She had many more men, and eventually another child—the one who just died. But, through this life, "she lost all interest in men" and had chosen celibacy. As had Toloki, in his ascetic life as a Professional Mourner.

Toloki visits Noria, and finds she has lost not only her son, but also her home, her shack in the squatter camp—or rather "informal settlement." With scrap materials from his friends, he helps her rebuild the shack in one night. She becomes interested in his work and joins him at a couple of funerals. He eventually becomes interested in her work, helping to care for orphans produced by the excess deaths of young parents. He is attracted to her, but remains reserved, formal, and professional. He is helping her because she is a homegirl from his village. She, for her part, has become less stuck-up since their teenage years, more mellow. She sees something profound in this odd comedic mourner.

After rebuilding the shack, she asks why he arrived by taxi instead of the cheaper trains. He says the trains are dangerous. "He has a mission in the world" he tells her, "that of mourning for the dead. It is imperative that he does his utmost to stay alive, so that he can fulfill his sacred trust, and mourn for the dead."[4] She is drawn to the passion for life in this oddball; she invites him to live with her: "I like you because you know how to live. I can teach you other ways of living."[5]

He demurs: "I cannot live with anyone but myself. That's why I decided to live alone in waiting rooms. That's why I decided not to have anything to do with homeboys and homegirls. I am a monk, Noria. A man with a vocation. I mourn for the dead. I cannot stop mourning, Noria. Death continues every day. Death becomes me, it is part of me.... I cannot live without death, Noria."[6]

But he reconsiders. He is drawn to her—yes, because she is beautiful, but mostly because she too "knows how to live." A night later he cannot sleep. He walks all night, pushing his shopping cart to her shack, and he moves in. The first night they are together, he looks at her sleeping and wants to hold her in his arms. "But of course he cannot do such a thing. He can't look at her sleeping posture for too long either. That would be tantamount to raping her."[7] In fact never, at least by the end of the book, does their mutual life-giving become sexual.

What is going on here? What is the point of mourning—especially Toloki, who does not even know the people he mourns for? What is mourning, if not feeling sad because we can't help it, and moving on as quickly as possible? Isn't it better to spend all that energy trying to solve the problem? Wouldn't it be more efficient to cut short the crying and get right to political negotiations or AIDS education?

And how can mourning be life-giving?

Mourning is remembering sorrowfully; in Greek it is *penthos*, related to *patho*, suffering. When we remember sorrowfully, we carry the pain—the literal meaning of suffering. Any time life is lost or diminished, we remember that life sorrowfully; it is natural, but it is also necessary. "Blessed are they that mourn," says the beatitude. "He who mourns his beloved one cannot be stopped" says the Kenyan proverb. The pain is there, and it must be carried. Likewise with suffering: we must be very careful in our efforts to "relieve suffering". We should seek to relieve affliction and pain, yes, but we dare not try to relieve a person of their *suffering*, their ability to carry the pain. Much better it is to have compassion—to suffer with, to mourn.

But what if there is too much pain? What if one person, or one family, or one nation, or one continent has too much pain to carry? Toloki knew that Africa had too much pain. He knew that he had to mourn for his own sake—"My body needs to mourn"[8]—but also for the sake of the nation. The pain had to be carried; it would not just go away. Toloki purified himself—at least to the point of not contributing to the political violence or AIDS spread, the most prevalent ways of dying—and then offered himself to come along side those who were mourning and, by mourning with them, help carry the load. Noria too, herself a victim of political violence, does not seek revenge; she too has purified herself and will not contribute to the ordinary ways of dying; she too is helping to carry the load in her caring for the orphans.

But what they *don't* do—spread violence and disease, and what they *do*—care for the orphans, are ironically only the background requirements and side effects of mourning. It's true: "our ways of living are our ways of dying," and those ways of living need to be purified. But also: "our ways of dying are our ways of living."[9]

Death *is* part of us; we cannot live without it. To live, and live fully, means getting close enough to death to see it in myself; to cry because I too am dying and may even be part of the reason for others' deaths.

Of course I will cry if I consider my own death, especially if it seems imminent. But how could I be part of the reason for the deaths from AIDS in Africa? During a discussion in Nairobi about AIDS in Africa, some friends suggested that one reason for the AIDS spread in Africa is a loosening of traditional moral codes and their replacement by Western values such as promiscuity—the "nihilistic playfulness" Katongole wrote about. My daughter Elizabeth was at the discussion and said little. Later, however, she connected this "playfulness" with the ethical framework of people in her generation, and wondered to what extent their values were being "exported" by the media to Africa. And if they were being exported, did that mean she and her friends bore some responsibility for the prevalence of AIDS in Africa? Mourning is not just carrying someone else's pain and death; it is admitting my own—and my part in the responsibility for others'.

But seeing "my" pain does not make mourning a solitary activity. Mourning must be corporate, say the African proverbs: "One person weeping prevents all in the village from sleeping." "When the eye weeps it makes the nose weep too." The entire living community carries the pain—it is our pain, our death. The entire living community: that means, in our global village, that we in the West are part of the same human community as Africa; that if they are the eye, we are the nose; that their weeping should keep us from sleeping.

So what does it mean for us to mourn for African AIDS? Is it reading a newspaper article with a picture of a horribly skinny woman lying in a mud hut with an emaciated big-eyed infant sucking from her flat wrinkled breast? Is it that we perversely cannot take our eyes off the picture? Is it when we read that she died hours after the picture was taken, and the infant the next day, all because (according to the journalist) neither had access to "life-saving" antiretroviral drugs—and we feel sad and angry and powerless? Is that mourning?

No, none of that makes a connection between them and me: between their humanity and my humanity, their pain and my pain, their poverty and my wealth, their deaths and my death. The newspaper article only reinforces how different they are from us. We don't mourn and carry their pain. Instead we become incensed that the world is so unjust—or are secretly and guiltily relieved that we are not that way. Or both. We want to act; we don't know how to act. Our empathetic energies get drained off in anger at pharmaceutical companies or corrupt African leaders or the backward African society.

This is not mourning: we are not carrying their pain. We don't know how to carry their pain because we have never made the connection between their pain and our pain, their humanity and our humanity. The closest we come is to affirm that if the drugs are available to us, they should be available to them—and this sentiment we call compassion. All of the good that we try to do for them—the transfer of money, technology, education, goods—we call compassion. And all of this "good" is our way of making them like us, so that their humanity becomes like our humanity, and their pains become like our pains. We make the connection between our humanities on *our* terms, and then bemoan the difference. And we call this compassion.

Africa neither needs nor wants this kind of "compassion". "The dream of Africa is to be its own subject.... What Africa desires now is the chance to be itself, in the sense of shaping its own future. A little help from friends... will doubtless be needed. But the vision and application of principles to reality will be, in the main, Africa's own."[10] We cannot decide what this "little help" should be based on our inadequate understanding of Africa, and certainly not based on our excess or what will be profitable to us—the current foundations of foreign aid. We can come a step closer to knowing what this little help should be by listening to Africa, which is the point of this book. We can approach the same understanding by being compassionate.

Real compassion, as we saw above, is "suffering with"; it is carrying the pain, it is mourning. We need to return to this original meaning of compassion, not because it fixes things, any more than Toloki fixed the problem of too much dying. We need to suffer with people in Africa because, until we do, we will never know how to help. Toloki's profession was not to stop the pain, but to admit that it was there, and carry it. This is the essence of compassion; any good that we try to do must start there.

How do we do this, we who live in the West? I cannot tell you how; for me it involves returning to Africa. But I can say this: we in the West are too much like the "people who pride themselves on being virtuous and despise everyone else" (Luke 18:9-14). The Pharisee, praying to himself, thanked God that he was not like the sinful tax collector, and then rattled off all the good he had done. But it was the tax collector who found favor with God; he admitted he had done wrong. Perhaps, to paraphrase that tax collector, what we need is simply to say, "God, be merciful to me, a human."

173

REFERENCES

[1] **Mda, Zakes (1995)**, *Ways of Dying* (Oxford, Oxford University Press), p.19-20.

[2] **Mda**, *Ibid.*, **1995** p. 7.

[3] **Mda**, *Ibid.*, **1995**, p. 11-12.

[4] **Mda**, *Ibid.*, **1995**, p. 96.

[5] **Mda**, *Ibid.*, **1995**, p. 115.

[6] **Mda**, *Ibid.*, **1995**, p. 115.

[7] **Mda**, *Ibid.*, **1995**, p. 153.

[8] **Mda**, *Ibid.*, **1995**, p. 150.

[9] **Mda, Ibid.**, **1995**, p. 98.

[10] **Magesa, Laurenti (2002)**, *Christian Ethics in Africa* (Nairobi, Acton Publishers), p.115.

INDEX

Printed in the United Kingdom
by Lightning Source UK Ltd.
120579UK00002B/150